Stephen Turoff

PSYCHIC SURGEON

Stephen Turoff

PSYCHIC SURGEON

The Story of an Extraordinary Healer

GRANT SOLOMON

Thorsons
An Imprint of HarperCollins*Publishers*

The Publishers regret that due to circumstances be-
yond their control they have not been able to trace or
acknowledge the copyright holder of Sathya Sai Baba
photograph. They will be happy to acknowledge the
photographer in future editions if they are notified.

Thorsons
An Imprint of HarperCollins*Publishers*
77–85 Fulham Palace Road
Hammersmith, London W6 8JB
1160 Battery Street
San Francisco, California 94111–1213

Published by Thorsons 1997

1 3 5 7 9 10 8 6 4 2

A catalogue record for this book
is available from the British Library

ISBN 0 7225 3461 2

Printed and bound in Great Britain by
Creative Print and Design (Wales), Ebbw Vale

For Dad

CONTENTS

ACKNOWLEDGEMENTS

A great many people have contributed to the making of this book. I would like to acknowledge all those who gave or sent me information, shared their experiences or generally encouraged or helped in whatever small way. Not all the detail and stories could be shared with the reader in this short book, but those not included are no less important to the final result.

I would especially like to mention my wife Jane and Stephen's wife Kathy for their contributions – Jane for her total support every step of the way and Kathy for her prodigious feats of memory and the many cups of tea, Sunday lunches, dinners and late night snacks that seemed to be such a feature of researching into the life and times of one of the world's most unusual living men, her husband Stephen.

INTRODUCTION

Stephen Turoff is a contemporary healer, teacher, priest, philosopher, knight, philanthropist and mystic. For a quarter of a century he has been healing people, by the tens of thousands, of all colours, castes and creeds. They flock from the four corners of the world to see him at his Danbury Healing Clinic near Chelmsford in Essex. For some, the journey is a pilgrimage; for others, a last chance to be healed. For most, it is an experience which will not be quickly forgotten.

Journalists, scientists, politicians, doctors and holy men of many faiths have had to admit that there is certainly something 'different' about this jovial, gentle giant with his gruff voice and permanent cheeky grin. When Stephen works, beautiful pastel lights descend like lightning bolts from the sky into patients' bodies, sacred ash forms on objects and people in his surgery, towels and sheets turn pink, and messages, finger-written in orange ochre, appear on photographs of saints. But most importantly, in many, many cases, the blind regain sight, the deaf hear, the lame cast away their crutches, diseased organs literally disappear and the sick and suffering are granted relief.

Who is this man who can work such wonders? He is a 16-stone, six-and-a-half foot, middle-aged Jewish-Christian former carpenter from Brick Lane in London's East End whom many believe to be an instrument of God. His message can be summed up in just four words: 'Love all, serve all.' But if you would like to know a little more, read on, for here is the strange but true tale of Stephen Turoff, psychic surgeon.

1

MEETING THE MYSTIC

Men occasionally stumble over the truth. But most pick themselves up and hurry off as if nothing happened.

WINSTON CHURCHILL

I met Stephen at a function in Holborn, London. It was 7 January 1989. I was one of 30 people sitting down to dinner. To my right was a grey-haired businessman. To my left, a very warm, outgoing and jovial giant of a man in his early forties whose accent was unmistakably East End. We shook hands and I learned that his name was Stephen Turoff. In many ways, he was larger than life. His physical presence was hard to ignore. But there was another presence, too, a sort of 'aura' which was coming at me in waves. I had no idea at the time, but this meeting was to change my life.

I made polite conversation.

'What do you do for a living?' was my imaginative best.

'I'm a parapsychologist,' he answered, casually. Oh brilliant, I thought, that's my subject too! Apparently sensing my unease, he immediately continued, 'Bit of a conversation stopper that one, isn't it?'

'Yes, I suppose it is. Um, what exactly do you mean?'

'Well, I take part in, research and investigate paranormal phenomena, especially psychic healing, and I've recently published a book about it.'

'Oh right,' I nodded.

Throughout dinner I also chatted to the man on my right. He told me he had first met Stephen at his clinic in the Barbican, London. To my surprise, this mature, reasonable businessman recounted how Stephen had slit his stomach open with a knife – but no anaesthetic – and had removed some 'diseased tissue' with his fingers, all in about 10 minutes. I then learned that other people around the table had also been to see this man they called the 'psychic surgeon' and many had experienced similarly incredible treatments.

I decided to investigate further. Collaring Stephen in the bar after dinner, I started asking the questions he must have heard so often before: 'What do you do? How does it work?' Having answered my initial barrage with some rather unbelievable brief answers, he proceeded to intrigue me further.

'I hope you don't mind me saying,' he whispered, gesturing to the barmaid, 'but I think you'll find you've forgotten your bus fare.'

The young woman was not at all convinced, until she checked her purse and found it empty!

'How did you know that?' I asked Stephen.

'Well, that's a longer story than we have time for this evening,' he answered cryptically and proceeded to change the subject.

When we were ready to leave, I asked if I could bring my youngest brother, Tom, along to the clinic which Stephen ran with his wife Kathy from their modest home in Danbury, Essex.

In the event, it was to be many months before I found myself pulling up, with my sceptical mother and apprehensive brother, outside the small but comfortable cottage-style, ex-council house.

We found ourselves in a crowded room with about 10 other people. Nearly everybody had either a wheelchair, crutches or bandages. Another 20 or so people who could stand unaided did so in a disorderly queue down the garden path. Not a business that makes for easy relations with the neighbours, I thought to myself. The four loudly ticking clocks, flower-patterned sofas and antique darkwood furniture added to the strange, almost spooky atmosphere.

Then a door was flung open and Stephen stormed past in a white coat. Well, I thought it was Stephen. But his wrinkled face looked a good 20 years older. He was round shouldered, as if slightly hunched, and he dragged his right leg along behind him as he rushed past us towards his wife, who was standing in the kitchen. He was physically smaller, enough to necessitate rolling his trousers up a couple of folds. I smiled to myself, wondering what my friends would make of it all, but came back to the room with a jolt when he spoke.

'I have told you not to leave the bits in the sink,' he barked at Kathy in a distinctly German accent.

'Sorry, Dr Kahn,' said Kathy apologetically and proceeded to clear out the sink. 'The bits' looked like the uncooked scraps you might throw the dog after preparing the Sunday roast.

'Dr Kahn' shuffled back into his operating room with another victim in tow and left my mother, brother and I looking at each other in disbelief.

'Look, Mum, we're here now so we might as well give it a go,' I said as persuasively as my own doubts would allow. She cautiously agreed and we stood around for another half an hour or so until it was Tom's turn. I went in with him.

'Good day to you,' the surgeon greeted us. 'My name is Dr Kahn. There is no death and I am living proof of that. Ha, ha.'

Oh great, I thought, a spirit with a sense of humour. That's all we need. But then it all got very serious. He laid my young brother down on the operating table and gently placed his hands on the chest area, without enquiring as to the problem.

In fact Tom suffered with asthma. Ten minutes later, it was all over.

'Well?' enquired my mother.

'Wasn't much to it,' said Tom nonchalantly, 'but his hands did get boiling hot, as hot as the radiator at home.'

We went home, wondering whether it was all a show, mass hypnotism or, worse, a gigantic, sustained, daily con. And to what end? Being an eighties-style materialist, I, of course, considered the financial angle. But there were a lot of easier ways to make money. I decided to leave the whole thing open and for the next few months got on with running my business.

However, a seed had been sown. I can only speak from personal experience but I believe it is impossible to meet Stephen Turoff without being affected in some way. It makes you think more deeply about health, life and death, and your 'reason for being' in general. For me, it was as if a switch had been flicked and the light illuminated a whole new world of possibilities, a world I had never imagined could exist.

I began to find out as much as possible about what was going on at that little house in Danbury. First of all, I learned about Dr Kahn and Stephen's other friends and helpers from what they call 'the life after Earth'. This is an alternative reality where time, space, matter and energy operate according to different laws. Apparently we are all destined to visit it. It is where Stephen's team continue their healing mission.

DR KAHN

Dr Joseph Abraham Kahn is a medical doctor. Sick people visit him from all over the world. His patients report that he performs many types of surgery, including neurosurgery, eye surgery and heart surgery; he manipulates their bones; he removes and replaces their organs; he makes their minds and

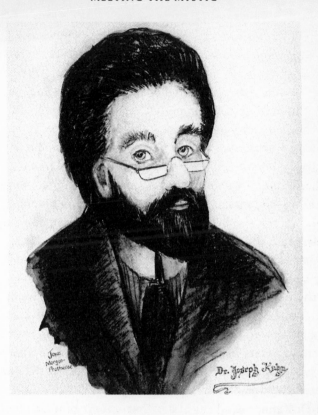

Joyce
Morgan-
Protheroe

Dr. Joseph Kahn

bodies well. There are numerous reports of his unorthodox methods resulting in miraculous cures. Dr Kahn died in 1912 ...

However, he tells us that it was simply a transition to another world. He arrived in 'another place, to the sound of my mother singing like a nightingale upon an evening's dusk':

It was a great surprise to me, to find myself alive when I was supposed to be dead. It is a lot for the rational mind to understand. If I could have one experience of my Earth life again, it would be my passing. When I met my mother, it was a beautiful, beautiful reunion. We hugged and there were tears. I had been a very material man on Earth and had not had much time for thoughts of God. My mother explained some truths to me. She said, 'Come, Joseph, come.' I was taken to a beautiful place. If you try to imagine the most beautiful place on Earth and double it, then you will have some appreciation of the place I was taken to. My world is very beautiful. I would not want to come back to Earth to live but I do want to help people in your world who are sick and troubled. I love people. I love my work. Love is the message I bring to you all from my world.

Today Dr Kahn is a 'spirit surgeon'. Whilst on Earth, he tells us that his medical techniques were fairly primitive – 'In my day, it was cut it out or cut it off!' – but since leaving the Earth the good doctor has learned much. He attended the 'Halls of Learning' on the astral planes and kept abreast of medical developments on Earth at the same time by visiting Earth hospitals in his spirit form. Apparently he also keeps himself acquainted with the work of other spirit surgeons around the world.

Dr Kahn now exists at a higher state of vibration than we do. So in order to function on what he calls 'the Earth plane' he must take over and use the body of a person who is still at our lower state of vibration. This is where Stephen Turoff comes in. Dr Kahn tells us that Stephen has been chosen 'for his strengths and not his weaknesses'. In order to use Stephen's body, Dr Kahn lowers his own state of vibration by the power of conscious thought. This enables him to take over Stephen's body and wear it much like a suit of clothes. As he explains:

In actual fact it's more like wearing a suit of armour. You see, my instrument is nearly six-and-a-half feet tall. My physical stature, when I was on Earth, was a

whole foot less than that. So when I lower my vibra-
tion to become as I was on the physical Earth plane,
I find it very difficult to step into and control such a
large body as Stephen's.

Vibration appears to be very important. We already know
that the same material, vibrating at different rates, can exist
in vastly different forms. Water, for example, can be a solid,
a liquid or a gas. Different vibrational rates could explain
many things: how ghosts move through walls; the appearance of saints and deities; hands and scalpels passing
through 'solid' flesh without breaking the skin during psychic surgery and a whole range of other phenomena, such as
milk-drinking statues, for example. Further investigation
into vibration might even throw some light on crop circles
and UFO sightings.

Thought energy is apparently very important in the spirit
world. Spirit beings, we are told, use thought to create objects
there. The vibration of the object is then lowered so that it
manifests or materializes in our world. The opposite effect
occurs when the spirit being raises the vibration of an object
and it 'disappears' or dematerializes.

If other worlds do operate on much higher vibrations or
frequencies than our own, they could occupy the same space
but not be visible, audible or tangible. You cannot see, hear or
touch the energy frequencies that transmit television signals
into your home – you only know they are there when you
turn on the receiver, the TV set. Is it going too far to suggest
that some human beings are naturally able to receive signals
from other worlds? Perhaps there might even be the possibility, in the future, of communication with these worlds, using
instruments designed specifically to pick up the signals for
those who do not have a natural capability.

There may even be the possibility of communication for

everybody today. We may all be capable of communicating with worlds which exist on other planes of vibration, but some of us do not know how to switch ourselves *on*. Alternatively, perhaps we switch ourselves *off* by allowing our 'rational' minds to block or interfere with the signals.

To go back to Dr Kahn, when he was on Earth he was a brown-eyed, black-bearded man with reading glasses and a limp. When he lowers his vibration and takes over Stephen's body, he appears to regain his disability and drags one leg behind him as he walks. He was also older than Stephen is now when he died. Consequently there are many reports that Stephen's face darkens and becomes the more wrinkled face of a much older man when he is entranced by Dr Kahn. I asked Stephen what it was like to be 'in trance':

> *Deep trance is like going to sleep. I don't remember anything about what has happened. The spirit helpers tell me they take me off to a beautiful place where I learn things. But I don't remember that either. It's like a sleep in which you never remember anything, not even your dreams. The human helpers and patients tell me what Dr Kahn did whilst I was gone.*

Dr Kahn tells us that he has a large team of 'spirit helpers':

> *I now have 17 assistants. My team consists of doctors, surgeons, healers and bone manipulators. We also have scientists who use their advanced knowledge of astral and physical science to bridge the gap between the dimensions and so make it all work.*

This concept of different dimensions may seem somewhat far-fetched. Yet scientists working in the field of what is sometimes called 'new physics' discuss them as a matter of course. Professor Stephen Hawking, in his bestseller *A Brief History of Time* (Bantam, 1988), explains as follows:

> *String theories, however ... seem to be consistent only if space-time has either ten or twenty-six dimensions, instead of the usual four! Of course, extra space-time dimensions are a commonplace of science fiction ...*
>
> *Why don't we notice all these extra dimensions ... why do we see only three space and one time dimension? The suggestion is that the other dimensions are curved up into a space of a very small size, something like a million million million million millionth of an inch. This is so small that we just don't notice it ... It is like the surface of an orange: if you look at it close up, it is all curved and wrinkled, but if you look at it from a distance, you don't see the bumps and it appears to be smooth. So it is with space-time: on a very small scale it is ten-dimensional and highly curved, but on bigger scales you don't see the curvature or the extra dimensions.*

So, though the rational mind boggles at the thought of 20 or so 'spirit people' beavering away in another dimension while in this one Stephen Turoff performs seemingly complex operations in minutes, it may well be possible.

NURSE GRACE

The foremost of Dr Kahn's helpers appears to be a woman who is known as Nurse Grace. There are more concrete details about her Earth life than about those of the other members of the team, including both a sketch drawing and a photograph of Grace. These have a fascinating history. Elsebe and Lloyd were South African patients and friends of the Turoffs who moved to Scotland from Ongar in Essex. They were invited to join the Spiritualist church in Aberdeen. In 1987 a psychic artist at the church, Len Lobban, was commissioned to do some portraits. He clairvoyantly 'saw' a woman standing beside Elsebe and drew her.

Clairvoyance is a French word which, taken literally, means 'clear seeing'. This might also be explained when we understand more about vibration. The 'normal' eye acts like a pinhole camera. It picks up the visible spectrum of light which is reflected off physical objects and the brain interprets the signals received and turns them into useful information. This is how we distinguish shape, texture, colour and so on. The visible spectrum is merely a limited range of vibrations or frequencies that most people can see. If some human beings are able to see a greater range of vibration, these 'clairvoyant' individuals might register more of what is going on around them than is the norm. The same goes for *clairaudience*, which means 'clear hearing'. We already know that bats, dogs and dolphins hear a wider range of sound than humans do. The ears and brains of clairaudient people may be better tuned to a range of vibrations or frequencies outside the normal spectrum. This would enable them, in theory, to 'hear' the voices of spirit people who are communicating using signals that other people simply do not hear.

Irrespective of how it works, Nurse Grace was visible to Len Lobban and, by some means, communicated her name. Elsebe did not recognize the person in the picture Len drew, but after giving it some thought, wondered whether the nurse was connected with Stephen Turoff and Dr Kahn. She sent the picture to the Turoffs, who questioned Dr Kahn about it. His answer was intriguing: 'Yes, it is Nurse Grace. She is one of our team. For now you have a drawing but, in the very near future, you will find a photograph of her as she was in her

Earth life.' Stephen and Kathy put the picture away and forgot all about it.

Eight months later, they were visiting the Mildmay Mission Hospital in the East End of London.

'As we entered the corridor,' Stephen told me, 'I noticed memorabilia of the hospital's past history on the walls. One picture stood out.' It was a likeness of Nurse Grace. Stephen made enquiries about the photograph, learned it was taken in 1893 and was given a copy of it. Nurse Grace had worked at the hospital nearly 100 years earlier. Now she was apparently back in spirit form, to continue her healing mission as one of Dr Kahn's team.

MR JAMES

In January 1990, Dr Kahn was giving a lecture and demonstration, through Stephen, at the Salon Varietes theatre in Fuengirola, Spain.

'My name is Dr Kahn, Joseph Abraham Kahn, and this is my assistant Mr R. James,' he announced, pointing to two portraits at the front of the stage. 'I am the good-looking one.' The audience laughed uncertainly.

Behind the portraits lies another fascinating story. They were painted by psychic Mijas resident Joyce Morgan-Protheroe, a freelance magazine illustrator, from images that 'simply appeared on paper' in front of her. She had no idea what Dr Kahn or Mr James looked like, nor had she any idea why they should be important. But when Stephen saw them on his visit to Spain, he was thrilled.

'That was the first time I had seen a picture of Dr Kahn, let alone Mr James,' he said. 'I have since been told that Mr James had a connection with King's College Hospital and that he died in the 1950s, but I haven't made enquiries. I have no need to know who these helpers were in their

Earthly incarnations. Others may want to know, but it makes no difference to me. It is the work they do now that is important.'

DR KAHN, JR

The first Dr Kahn is an elderly man whose temperament and characteristics belong firmly in the nineteenth century. Apparently he had a son, another surgeon called Dr Kahn, who is now also a spirit surgeon. This second Dr Kahn appears to be younger and more modern in temperament and character. We are told that he was a surgeon on the battle-fields of France during the First World War and that he was known for his willingness to treat all the wounded, from whatever side. He 'came through' to work with Stephen early in 1991. This second Dr Kahn's portrait was also drawn by Joyce Morgan-Protheroe. One French patient, a lady in her nineties, actually remembered him from the days of the Great War. She had a conversation with him about those terrible times and the memories so upset him that he had to leave Stephen's body for the afternoon and his father had to take over for the remainder of the session.

OTHER MEMBERS OF THE SPIRIT TEAM

Various other helpers have come through to use Stephen's body at different times. These include Professor Pafi, an Egyptian who describes himself simply as 'a healer', and Dr Gino, an Italian who has spoken to patients in both his own language and English. We believe, from the little that has been said, that Dr Gino may now be taking charge of the work in Spain. There have also been indications that the world-renowned Brazilian psychic surgeon José Arigo has recently joined the band of helpers. The rest of the team remain, as yet, anonymous.

I asked Stephen a question that might worry many people if they had his ability to go into trance: 'Aren't you ever scared that, because beings from another world have control of your body, anything could happen and you would be held responsible?'

Stephen answered, 'I have complete faith in God. Dr Kahn and his team are doing God's work. I have total faith in their motives and their methods.'

It seems that this faith is justified. There are literally tens of thousands of people who have testified to the effectiveness of whatever it is that Stephen, Dr Kahn and his team actually do during the healing process. At the Danbury Healing Clinic, the waiting room is full every day of the week. Ambulances bring people on stretchers and in wheelchairs. Coaches come from Wales once a fortnight. Less regularly, they arrive from Germany, France, Turkey and other places around the world. When Stephen attends his clinic in Spain, 1,000 people are treated during each 10-day trip. In his Israel clinic, he has treated as many as 177 patients in one day.

'You treat so many people. Has anything ever gone wrong?' I asked Stephen ... delicately.

'Now and then something regrettable happens. Once, somebody tripped me up by accident when I was in deep trance and I fell on the patient. The poor bloke was only small. With a big lump like me falling on him, he suffered cracked ribs. Luckily the patient and the person who tripped me up were friends, otherwise things might have got out of hand!'

2

THE FAMILY

Love begins at home ... but that isn't where it
ends.

REVEREND PETER NOKES

As I became fascinated with what was going on at the clinic, I
began to piece together the story of Stephen's life. It began
back in the summer of 1947...

Stephen was born at 1.50 p.m. on 26 July 1947, at South-
meads Hospital, Bristol. The 10lb wrinkly bundle of arms and
legs, nicknamed 'Winston Churchill' by the nurses, was the
third child and only son of Cyril and Kitty Turoff and new
baby brother to Evelyn, nine, and Sandra, nearly four.

The Turoff family originally came from Russia. Stephen's
great-great-grandfather, Shiar Turoff, had arrived in London in
the 1840s, a penniless refugee who had suffered anti-Semitic
persecution in his home country. He had four children, all boys:
Morris, Lewis, Tobias and Samuel. Tobias, Stephen's great-
grandfather, was born in 1846. He and his wife Minnie had
seven children: Rose, Annie, Barnet, Lewis, Simon, Stephen's
grandfather, who was born in 1890, Sidney and Marie. Some
left London and went off to America, the emerging land of
opportunity, to seek their fortunes, but Simon stayed and started work in 1904 as an apprentice cabinet maker. He later married Martha, a girl from Tower Hamlets. Cyril, born in 1912,
was the first of their five children and he was followed by Lily,
Sadie, Montague and finally Evelyn, who was born in 1921.

Stephen also had Russian blood on his mother's side. His maternal grandfather, Peter Leshinsky, born in 1890, was descended from landed Russian Cossacks, but his wife Mary, a seventh child, was from a wealthy family whose money had been made from trade. The perceived incompatibility between their aristocratic and middle-class backgrounds led to Peter and Mary leaving their home country in order to escape family recriminations. On arriving in London, Peter trained as a cabinet maker and invested in saw-mills. He and his wife had nine children, the seventh of whom was Katherine, Stephen's mother, who was known as Kitty from an early age. Some find it interesting that Kitty was the seventh child of a seventh child, as legend has it that such children have psychic abilities. Kitty certainly did have a psychic gift and performed readings which were very accurate – until she forecast a friend's death and never did it again.

During the 1920s, Peter Leshinsky began to drink to excess. Once he even managed to drink white horse liniment by mistake. He foamed at the mouth and, looking despairingly at 10-year-old Kitty, proclaimed, 'I'm dead, I'm dead in heaven and you're an angel.' In another incident, he tried to mend his severed finger by plunging it in a pot of glue. He ended his days living on his own in Gosset Street, just off Brick Lane.

So both sets of Stephen's grandparents lived in the East End of London and both families were in the business of cabinet making. However, there the similarities ended. One family was working-class and Jewish, the other middle-class and Christian. These differences were destined to cause no end of problems when Cyril, an upholsterer and a lovable rogue with a liking for the dog track, met Kitty in the mid 1930s.

At that time many top East End villains were employed by the fascist leader Oswald Mosely, there was anti-Semitic rioting in Whitechapel and for a short while Bethnal Green was known as 'the fascist manor'. The atmosphere was hostile. At the so-called 'Battle of Cable Street' on 11 October 1936, 100,000 people built barricades and poured out onto the streets in an attempt to prevent a march by 7,000 fascist supporters. Lorries were overturned, bricks thrown at the police and roads strewn with glass to prevent charges by mounted officers. Eighty people, including 15 policemen, were injured and there were 84 arrests. Regardless, six weeks later, on 28 November 1936, Cyril Turoff married Kitty Leshinsky at Bethnal Green Town Hall Registry Office.

A year or so later Evelyn was born. Then came the war. Cyril was posted around the country whilst he was training. While he was in Narbeth, north Wales, he was joined by his wife and young daughter, for they had been bombed out of London in the Blitz. Returning home from the air raid shelter one morning, Kitty had found a wasteland. The house had literally disappeared, along with the rest of the street.

Eventually Cyril was sent to Europe as a front-line motorbike dispatch rider. One day, in the pouring rain, he and his best friend had to get across some open fields to deliver urgent dispatches. They did not want to risk crossing the exposed ground and decided that the hedges alongside the fields would afford the best protection against snipers. In the noise and confusion of battle, Cyril's young friend, riding ahead, did not hear the approaching enemy tank which came straight through the hedge, crushing and severing both his legs. It is not difficult to imagine the profound effect this awful sight had on Cyril.

Asking for a transfer to different work, he was moved to front-line ambulance driver. This was equally harrowing. One of the jobs involved the clearing of the bodies and 'pieces' of his comrades from the battlefield in sacks and identifying them in whatever way possible. The Jews were especially difficult to identify as they carried neither papers nor tags in case of capture by the Nazis.

Towards the end of the war, Cyril was one of the first to enter a concentration camp. The SS guards had left in a hurry and, in a feeble attempt to cover up atrocities, had bulldozed hundreds of bodies under mounds of earth at the gates of the camp. On entering, a member of Cyril's unit noticed that the huge mounds were moving. Not all of the bodies were dead!

Cyril's war ended when he was driving over a bridge in a forest and a mortar round landed in his cab. He was lucky to be alive, but sustained terrible injuries and spent a long time as unidentified wounded in a Dutch hospital before eventually being shipped home. His brother Montague was to recall in a conversation with Stephen, some 50 years later, that Cyril was being carried from the battlefield with shrapnel lodged in his brain, as he, Monty, was going onto it.

Kitty and Evelyn had meanwhile been transferred from north Wales to a hut in a forest near Weston-super-Mare. Eventually they were moved to the home of 'a very religious Christian family who said prayers all the time', according to Evelyn. Sandra was born there and it was then decided that they should move in with Kitty's sister in Sand Bay, near Kewstoke, Weston-super-Mare. When the war ended, this arrangement became too crowded and so they moved on again, to a cottage in Cheddar. They were living there when Stephen was born, but finally, in 1948, moved back to Brick Lane.

As a child Stephen was destined to be almost constantly ill. When he was only two years old, a raging temperature would be followed by a coma-like state and a rush to hospital. These comas, at their worst, would occur as often as once a fortnight and continued for many years. This was the beginning of a living nightmare of debilitating illness followed by acute condition followed by minor sickness, and so on and so on. Much later, Stephen was to be told that his constant illness was part of his preparation for the healing of others.

Cyril, too, had recurring health problems. Shrapnel was still lodged in his brain and he would wake at night in terrible pain with blood oozing from his ears. Stephen slept in his parents' room and remembers his father up at night groaning with the pain. Later Cyril was to suffer from ulcerated legs which required long periods of time in the Mildmay Mission Hospital, Shoreditch. When healthy, he weighed 16 stones, but his prolonged suffering was to make him a shadow of his former self. He was often in hospital for a month or more at a time.

Kitty had to work hard. She tried out a range of jobs and for a time ran a paper stall near Liverpool Street. Then, in the early 1950s, she took over the restaurant in Virginia Road, Shoreditch, where she had once worked and it became known to all around as 'Kitty's'.

Although the union of Jew and Christian was frowned on by both families, Stephen remembers being allowed to see his Jewish grandmother, Martha, at Christmas and on his birthdays. 'She would give me a lovely moustache-smacker of a kiss and there was always another shilling for my money box.' This irregular contact between grandparent and child would not have been so unusual if they had been miles apart, but Martha actually lived upstairs in the same block of flats! Stephen has fond memories of his gran and wonders today what might have been if the family feud had been less intense. His Aunt Evelyn also lived upstairs; she did not have any time for 'silly feuds' and Stephen saw quite a bit of her.

In 1952, Stephen started at Virginia Road School, Shoreditch. He suffered from dyslexia, but not much was known about the condition then and, perhaps due in part to constant sickness and his unrecognized learning difficulty, Stephen became very much a loner. He was a nervous child who tried to mask his dyslexia with bad handwriting. In order to get the 'stupid' child out of the classroom as much as possible, the teachers assigned him jobs like milk monitor and litter boy. He was, however, very good at maths, having no trouble with mathematical symbols. At seven, he had mastered logarithms and anti-logarithms. He had a limited interest in sports, but enjoyed football, which he played for the school.

Stephen's sisters were very good to him. At the Coronation on 2 June 1953, he remembers them dressing him up as a sailor in raffia paper. With Dad unwell and Mum working, Evelyn and Sandra would really fuss over their little brother and were fiercely protective of him.

Yet although he had a loving, caring family, Stephen nevertheless experienced feelings of extreme loneliness. From the age of about six, he constantly imagined himself cradled in the arms of a 'Divine Mother'. He felt detached, as if he didn't quite belong in the world. He had 'an inner yearning to go home … to God, my other mum'. This highly unusual childhood affinity with God manifested in a love of listening to religious music of all kinds and a fascination with all religious stories, especially about the life of Jesus.

About a year after starting to think of God as his other mother, Stephen became aware of a lion 'panting and pacing around me'. In time of trouble, the lion would be there, he soon came to believe, to protect him. Others also saw and heard it from time to time. They reported catching a glimpse of the benevolent beast moving through a doorway or hearing it breathing behind furniture when Stephen was around. Much later, a superimposed image of a lion was captured on a photograph taken at Stephen's healing clinic in Chelmsford.

Around the same time Stephen also began to experience what he called the 'whispering shadows'. Voices would whisper around him and out of the corner of his eye he would catch sight of shadowy figures. To most children this would be very disconcerting, but Stephen belonged to a family of mystics who had some understanding of the unseen dimensions. As well as his mother, Stephen's sisters were both psychic, Evelyn so much so that she could clearly see people from the spirit world. When she married, she moved to a flat in a nearby block. The previous occupant, Mrs Chiswick, had recently died and Evelyn 'felt' the old lady there for a long time before she finally materialized one night and said, 'I'm looking for Sylvie. Do you know where my Sylvie is?' Evelyn had to explain to the old lady that her daughter Sylvie had moved to Dagenham.

'I thought it was all a lot of nonsense, when I was younger,' Sandra told me, 'but then a voice in my head said, "I will help you to believe, look up and you will see ..." So I looked up above my head and there was a kaleidoscope of faces all spinning round and grinning at me. Then lots of other unusual things started happening to me. When you have experiences like this, it's difficult not to believe.'

Cyril, meanwhile, liked a bet on the dogs. The small-time East End gambling scene attracted an array of eccentric people, including a notoriously flamboyant gent who called himself Prince Honolulu and had set himself up as a man who could accurately predict races for a fee. The Prince was absolutely huge. Of Hawaiian appearance, he wore three-foot feathers in a headband and conducted his business at the Shoreditch Church end of Brick Lane. He would strutt along the road shouting: 'I got a horse, I got a horse.' One day Prince Honolulu stopped, stooped down and, placing his large hand gently on young Stephen's head, asked Cyril: 'Do you realize who this boy really is?' Cyril brushed it off as the Prince's usual strangeness. But it may well have been that he was truly psychic and had seen something of what was to come.

At that time, normally when male Jews married Gentiles the children would be raised in the mother's faith. Stephen, however, was initially drawn to Judaism and attended what he called 'Jewish Sunday school'. This ended one summer sports day when, having won the first prize of a shilling in a race, Stephen was devastated to be slapped around the face by the rabbi, who said he must have cheated. So shocked was he that 'a so-called man of God' could do this that he never went back.

Meantime his health problems continued. At school, after assembly, the call would go out: 'Anyone for the clinic?' Whilst this service was intended to provide medical care for children in a deprived area, it also provided an ideal opportunity for a dyslexic, lonely child to get away from normal school for an hour or two. So Stephen would search his body for anything that might justify the clinic. When he was 10, however, he got more than he bargained for. Having found a very obliging lump on his knee, he was sent straight from the clinic to the Mildmay Mission Hospital. He had developed a cancerous growth. Stephen still vividly remembers the kindness of the Christian nurses in the hospital, 'always singing hymns'. Fortunately, an operation removed the tumour completely. This was typical of Stephen's childhood experience – lots of illness but always over it quickly. The next thing was glandular fever.

Later, when Stephen was 12, he entered what he describes as a 'very frightening' period, which lasted until he was 14. Lying in his bed at night, at the stroke of midnight, a tap, tap, tap on his forehead would awaken him. He would sit up with a start, trying desperately to catch a glimpse of his tormentor, but to no avail. Even if he stayed awake well into the night 'the tapper' would wait until he had just gone to sleep before playing his ghostly game. Then, two years after it had started, this one-sided wind-up stopped as abruptly as it had begun.

Stephen never found out whether it was a friendly spirit teasing him or something altogether more sinister.

Another 'very frightening' thing happened one afternoon when the whole family were out. Stephen was sick and went into his sisters' bedroom to sleep by snuggling into the feather bed. He awoke to hear a group of people chatting and partying in the living room. He tried to move but was frozen, as if held down by an unseen force. Eventually the noise subsided and he was able to move. Mustering all his courage, he ventured into the living room – to find there was nobody there.

From an early age, the young cockney was a bit of a showman. He would get jobs at the travelling fairs which pitched camp locally simply by hanging around Kitty's and asking the fairground operators for work. It was good holiday money and exciting and rewarding work. Stephen's favourite job was at the 'Wheel 'em' table:

> *Punters would roll a penny from one end of a specially designed table and the pennies would land on squares at the other end with numbers in them. The number in the box your penny landed in would decide the amount you won or didn't win. Believe it or not, at age 12, this was a really fun game table for me to be running and I made quite a few bob at it every year when the fairs came, until I was about 15, when these games lost some of their appeal.*

Stephen's natural talent for drawing crowds was noticed by Stevie Gray, a well known fairground operator. He offered the young crowd-pleaser a permanent job with the fair, but it was too much to contemplate, 'what with the travelling and being away from Mum and Dad', so Stephen decided against it.

It is interesting to speculate as to what might have been if he had chosen to accept Mr Gray's kind offer. Tens of thousands of people might not have had the benefit of his healing gift – or perhaps they still would have done. Perhaps, if it is our destiny or purpose to do certain things in our life, fate or chance or God will bring us back to them whatever decisions we might make along the way.

Early in 1960, aged 13, Stephen went into hospital for an appendix operation. Cyril was in the same ward. On the first night, the man in the next bed to Stephen passed peacefully away. The nurses thought Stephen might be upset and moved him to the end of the ward. On the second night, again the man in the next bed to Stephen passed away. The nurses moved Stephen to the other side of the ward. But on the third night the same thing happened. And on the fourth.

The young lad came to be feared as such a jinx that even Cyril considered whether it was advisable to be in the next bed. They moved Stephen to the middle of the ward with no one either side of him. A kindly old gentlemen was in the bed opposite and he comforted the confused young boy and told him not to worry about the strange coincidences. That night, he passed away quietly in his sleep.

The nurses refused to believe in jinxes but nevertheless decided that Stephen should have a screen around his bed for the peace of mind of the other patients. Stephen was later told by his spirit friends that each of his neighbours had been very sick and in great pain. His presence had, in some way, enabled their peaceful release.

The next year Stephen collapsed with suspected polio on a day trip to Southend. What started as a sunny day out ended with him being rushed to Rochford Hospital. Once again he recovered quickly, however, and was discharged a few days later. Some weeks afterwards, he was walking across a field and, hearing a warning shout, looked around to be struck by an arrow fired by another boy with a home-made bow. The arrow went in at the left side of the left eye, causing a haemorrhage and an injury which has left the eye partially closed to this day. Another two weeks in hospital followed.

When he was 15, Stephen 'put away childish things' and started work as a cabinet maker's apprentice. He was soon to have 'a lot' of girlfriends and has, ever since, especially enjoyed the company of women. 'Perhaps it's because the girls were a bit more sensitive and I felt very comfortable in their company,' he muses today, 'or perhaps it was more about discovering normal boy/girl attraction. I don't know. All I can say is, I really did enjoy going out and spending time with girls.'

The 'flicks', dancing at the Tottenham Royal and Flamingo night-clubs and hanging out at the Two Eyes coffee bar in the West End were some of the favourite activities of young people from Bethnal Green in the early sixties. Stephen remembers those times with special affection. Earning the princely sum of £3.10s.0d per week, he could just about afford both his bohemian social life and to pay something towards his keep.

Stephen had been associated with cabinet making from an early age. The owners and managers of local firms would come into Kitty's and would be ideal targets for his requests for weekend and holiday work. He was always prepared to work in order to get money and had long since learned the skills of a 'pesterer'. This, in East End parlance, means a 'buyer and seller of anything and everything'. The slightly brash young fairground showman was pretty good at it and was often occupied in activities like collecting comics for resale to other boys and 'raiding the bins for books and other toot 'n' tat' the market traders might give him a few pennies for.

From the start, the young apprentice had an affinity with wood:

I could make anything and everything and loved working with wood. It was alive to me. Consequently I got off to a really good start with the firm. Unfortunately, the persistent illness that has plagued my life reared its head again and I became so ill with various symptoms, including a raging temperature, that I was confined to bed for weeks and they had to let me go.

On recovering from this mystery illness, Stephen secured a job as an electrician's mate. To this day, he still has no idea why he chose this unfamiliar work. He did not enjoy it at all. He stuck at it for a year until, on turning 17, an opportunity came up as a carpenter with Illet and Wake, a small firm of builders' merchants who were trusted by the jewellers in Hatton Garden and consequently did a lot of work there. It was whilst working for Illet and Wake that Stephen had his first 'entity experience' away from home.

It happened when he was working with another carpenter making bookcases for what was to be a library for overseas students of economics in a large Georgian house in west London. At the end of the first week, the Irish caretaker of the house pulled the young apprentice to one side. 'Could you be doing with a little extra work at the weekend, lad?' This involved dismantling some of the old metal bookcases in the basement hallway and transporting the books up flights of stairs to their new home almost at the top of the house. So Stephen found himself rolling up early on the Saturday morning at the mansion.

After a cup of tea the caretaker went out shopping with his wife and for the first hour or so, all was well. Then

Stephen had just placed some books on the shelves in one of the library rooms when a thud, thud, thud went across the ceiling. Heart racing, Stephen tiptoed, hammer clasped in trembling fist, to the top landing and gingerly pushed open the door. 'Whew, no one there,' he sighed with relief. Nevertheless, just to make sure, he conducted a thorough search and checked that the top floor window was locked from the inside.

Still jittery, he descended to the slightly cramped and ill-lit basement area. In this dark subterranean den, the Irishman and his wife had made a comfortable home with a kitchen, living room and bedroom. From the hallway at the bottom of the stairs all three rooms were visible through their glass doors. Balancing on a small three-step ladder, Stephen began to dismantle the metal bookcases lining the hall.

Suddenly a blood-curdling yell came from the kitchen. Stephen whirled round, nearly toppling from the ladder. Hammer raised once more, he flung open the kitchen door and rushed in to find ... an eerie silence. The air was thin and a chilling stillness sent shivers up Stephen's spine. Nervously he went back to work, taking care to close the kitchen door securely. But within minutes, he heard somebody walking down the stairs.

'Oh good, you're back at la ...' he began, turning to greet the caretaker. But there was no one there. Still the footsteps continued down the stairs and then, rooted to the spot, Stephen felt icy breath in his right ear. Up in the air went the hammer and up the stairs went the apprentice, straight out of the front door and down the street as fast as his long legs could carry him.

Around the corner, Stephen found sanctuary in a café and sympathetic, if slightly sceptical, comfort from the plump, middle-aged lady behind the counter. 'A cuppa and a bun should do the trick,' she said. But it would take more than

tea and cake to get the strapping youth back in that basement. He waited a full two hours outside the house for the
return of the caretaking couple and told them the story from
start to finish.

'Oh beejaesus!' said the Irishman.

'Oh beejaesus!' said the Irishman's wife.

'Precisely!' said the young cockney.

Thankfully, there was not much more left to do and
Stephen managed to finish the job by the end of the day – but
only after insisting that someone kept him company at all
times.

After this, Stephen began to have many more unusual
experiences and encounters. One of the most common was
seeing 'people' standing next to people. Objects would move
without physical contact from any person. Coloured lights
would dance and jitter around everyone he looked at. Stephen
began to wonder if his mind was quite right.

Still, he was enjoying life, especially in the company of
Jean, a girl he had met at the Tottenham Royal. She was fair-
haired, good-natured, attractive and intelligent. Six months
Stephen's junior, she worked as a legal secretary. As the relationship developed they began to spend more and more time
together.

The following year, having just turned 18, Stephen fell ill
yet again, this time with what the hospital called 'a tropical
disease'. This was a little unexpected since he had never left
Britain! Throughout the first night in hospital, it was touch
and go as to whether he would survive and he was given 32
injections. Stephen says he remembers the 'very big needle'
vividly, but I was told by his sisters that he appeared completely delirious when admitted to hospital and remained that
way for quite some time. It was not until a full year later that
his mother felt able to tell him that they had nearly lost him
that first night.

It has since been explained to Stephen that his personal trauma, pain and suffering have been necessary to 'soften his heart' to the suffering of others. However, just like the rest of us, Stephen may also be travelling his own karmic path back to God. Perhaps there are karmic debts to pay along the way. Some speculate that, at our highest level of eternal being, we 'choose' our difficult earthly experiences in order to get back on the right road home to God, a road from which we might have strayed in former lives. Others say that there is no such thing as reincarnation or karma and that this is the only life-time we are granted, so we must get it right ... or else. Stephen himself is certain that the all-knowing, all-loving God in whom he has total faith would not allow the unneces-sary and undeserved suffering of any one of his children. Whatever the real truth, for him, it is enough to be convinced that 'God knows best'.

In 1966, after an 18-month courtship, Stephen married Jean at Hackney Town Hall. They moved into a small Bethnal Green flat and in a very short time encountered problems with bur-glars. While still doing his apprenticeship as a carpenter and joiner, Stephen was dealing in jewellery in order to generate a second income. This might have come to the attention of local thieves, for the newlyweds were burgled three times in the space of six months. One night Stephen actually saw a pair of eyes peering through the letterbox as a gang surveyed their next job.

Soon he found more extra work in the evenings as a door-man at the Lyceum Ballroom. The other bouncers nicknamed the cuddly giant 'Yogi Bear'. He also did other jobs in his 'pen-guin suit', as he called it, including an evening as personal bodyguard for an MP. Other jobs included being the back-door guard at the Miss World competition.

On another occasion, Stephen was patrolling the Lyceum dance floor and having a lark with some of the guests when an attractive girl came up to him, looking very pale.

'I'm June. I've lost my friend Carol,' she said and went on to describe Carol in detail. Must be a bit tipsy, thought Stephen to himself. Then he noticed a girl fitting Carol's description.

'Are you Carol?'

'Yes.'

'Your friend June's looking for you,' said Yogi Bear, 'and she doesn't look well.'

Carol's reaction was quite unexpected. She was so shocked that she had to be helped off the dance floor and began crying uncontrollably. June had died in an accident three weeks before! Stephen quickly made himself scarce.

Whilst in lots of ways he enjoyed dealing in a bit of jewellery and doing jobs in the penguin suit, Stephen could not get away from the objects moving around him, the voices calling his name and from the incredible visions of himself as a very religious man. The part he was playing in life was somehow alien. He knew he was searching for something, something more. But what was it? During his early twenties, the spiritual awakenings within him grew more pronounced and he started to have a series of what he calls 'personal spiritual experiences', developing an 'emotional need for God to come into my life'.

For the time being, however, it was Stephen's first child, Jason, who came into his life. It was 1969 and Stephen was working in Hatton Garden. When he got news that Jean was in hospital, he jumped into his van and raced off without any thought for the speed limit. Hurtling down Hackney Road in a rusty and battered old Ford Thames was just asking for trouble. When Stephen screeched to a halt at the red lights, an arm in a dark blue tunic came through the open window and five huge fingers landed on his shoulder. A grey-haired policeman put his nose right up to Stephen's face.

'Do you know what I'm going to have you for, sonny? Speeding and dangerous driving – and that's just the start of it!'

'My wife's just been rushed into hospital,' blurted Stephen, 'I'm going down there to see her having our baby.'

Luckily, the policeman was sympathetic. 'Well, be careful you don't make your child an orphan then!'

On arrival at the hospital, Stephen discovered it was all a false alarm. But Jean had nearly lost the baby and the doctors kept her in for the next five weeks as a precaution. Jason was eventually born with more than a few complications and a little jaundiced, but otherwise healthy. Stephen and Jean took him home to Bethnal Green. Just five weeks later, they moved to Witham in Essex.

The late sixties were a time of exodus to Essex for many from the East End. Towns like Harlow and Romford were generally the favoured destinations, but Stephen preferred the idea of moving a little further out. A comfortable three-bedroomed terraced council house in Poplar Close, Witham, looked like paradise to the young couple from the inner city.

Moving wasn't without its problems, however. In common with many young men, Stephen had not been lucky with motor vehicles. His current mode of transport was a blue (and brown if you include the rust) Ford Thames van. Coughing and spluttering along, this poor thing tried to transport them to Witham, but, hopelessly overloaded, gave up the ghost on the A12. They had to thumb a lift to Chelmsford, hire another van, drive back to the Ford Thames, unload its contents into the second van and tow the first to the nearest garage mechanic, who then took a further few hours to get it repaired …

In spite of all this, Stephen was very excited about the prospects ahead.

3

DEVELOPMENT:
THE 'HANDS-ON' HEALER

It's good to be a seeker, but sooner or later you
have to be a finder. And then it is well to give
what you have found, a gift into the world for
whoever will accept it.

JONATHAN LIVINGSTON SEAGULL

The move from London to Witham marked the arrival of a
new baby daughter, Nicole, and was also a time of intensifying spirituality for Stephen. He became much more aware
that he wanted to follow a deeply spiritual path in life, even if
he was still unsure as to what it was or how to go about it.
What pointed him in the next direction, as is so often the
case, was the death of a loved one – his father, Cyril.

Whilst Stephen felt that this was a welcome release from
years of suffering, it was nevertheless a terrible blow to lose
'my old dad'. The funeral took place in Hackney Road on 16
March 1972. Back in Colchester, Stephen chanced to look up
when passing a poster outside a Spiritualist church. Intrigued,
he carefully noted down the time of the service but still managed to arrive late on the day. Tentatively opening the door, he
encountered 40 or so people inside singing hymns.

Just another church, probably not for me, he thought to
himself but something prompted him to enter. Finding an
empty chair, he was surprised to experience 'a wonderful
warmth' as soon as he sat down. 'It felt as if I was in the right

place, spiritually, for the first time in my life. The only way to describe it is like "coming home".'

Stephen did not know what to expect next. In front of him, on a rostrum, were a man and a woman. The man appeared to be running the proceedings and it soon became apparent that the lady was a guest speaker and medium. She gave a talk for about 20 minutes on spirituality and then gave a demonstration of clairvoyance.

Thinking that no one had noticed him, Stephen was very surprised to be singled out when she pointed to him and said, 'This is the first time you've been to a Spiritualist church. Your guides have been waiting for you to make up your mind and to take some positive action. You've been on the fence for some time now. They couldn't do much until you jumped off. You've done that by coming here today. There is a very wise Chinese gentleman standing by you. He says his name is Chan. You will be doing great things if you can apply yourself. Chan is telling me that when he is ready to work with you, he will take off his cap and place it on your head. He will not be ready until you have made yourself ready. You have to apply yourself and make some progress before he will transfer his cap.'

Stephen travelled home very excited by this experience. It had been somewhat unsettling, though, and he is not sure what made him go back the next week. But he liked the way he was treated and the fact that, for the first time in his life, he felt at home in a spiritual environment: 'The cup of tea and biscuits atmosphere of the place was a big plus and I just felt drawn to the whole idea.'

He decided to learn how to meditate and began to read anything he could get his hands on to do with spiritual matters. Soon he found that he seemed to know a lot of it by instinct anyway. He set aside a period of time each and every day to meditate. He would go into his bedroom at 6 p.m. every night and sit quietly with his eyes closed. 'It was much like falling asleep.' He would then awaken at exactly 7.20 p.m. and go and have his dinner. He did this every day of the week, including weekends, for a whole year.

Almost immediately, a much wider range and intensity of phenomena began to happen around him. He learned at the Spiritualist church that, as he put it, 'God is like electricity and people are like light bulbs. When you decide to plug your-self in, the light comes on. The more often you plug yourself in, the brighter becomes the light.'

During this early period of intensifying phenomena, Jean also had some experiences and it turned out that she, too, was very sensitive to the spirit world. One night, she saw a bright glow in the corner of the bedroom. Out of the glow formed a mist. Out of the mist came a Native American who 'did some-thing to Stephen's head' while he slept. This particular event became a regular occurrence and once Jean even reported see-ing the Native American take Stephen out of his body and dis-appear with him as they both walked away into the mist.

Stephen was told that the phenomena were his 'carrots', signs that he was on the right path. He kept on going back to the church and received different messages each week to encourage and guide him. One day, a visiting medium whom he had never met before told him some very intriguing things from the rostrum.

'Did you know you could be a great healer? I have a Chi-nese gentleman with you who is taking off his cap and placing it on your head. He tells me there are big plans for you if you choose the healing path. Does this mean anything to you?'

The messages that followed told Stephen that he was ready to start healing and gave some pointers. Then, with the help of the people at the church, 'I just started putting my hands on people and asking God to help them.'

By now, at the age of 25, Stephen was established in Witham with a wife, two children, a house and a car. He had worked up to the responsible job of foreman joiner and effectively ran a small joinery works. His duties involved supervising new jobs and one day he had to go to the Corn Exchange in London to check some refurbishment work. Whilst standing in one of the rooms there he felt an incredible energy surge, his arms were lifted up and he was physically raised several inches off the ground. At first he was very scared, but this and other phenomena became more regular. It was then that people around Stephen began noticing that there was something 'different' about him.

In 1974, Stephen's second daughter, Zoë, was born. A few months later, having been hands-on healing for about two years, his ability was recognized as special for the first time. A local girl, nine-year-old Lynne Saunders, had been diagnosed as having a rare form of cancer. After operations in Chelmsford and extensive tests and radiation treatment in London, she was undergoing specialist drug treatment. A friend suggested to her mother, Carol, that she should take Lynne to see Stephen at his home. Mrs Saunders admitted her initial scepticism to Eve Sweeting of the local *Witham Evening Gazette*:

I was as sceptical as most people about spiritual healing. I went to see Stephen with Lynne. At that time, after her hospital treatments, she was thin, felt the cold a lot and had lost all her hair. I knew that children in her ward had died. But all the doctors were marvellous and we have nothing but praise for them. Stephen gave her a tremendous amount of help with spiritual healing. There was nothing to be afraid of. He just laid his hands on Lynne.

'His hands felt hot on me,' Lynne said. 'After seeing him every week I began to feel really well. I put on weight and my hair gradually started to grow again, far better than before. I stopped feeling cold all the time.' Just before Christmas, she was told that her illness was in a state of remission. She stayed well and by 1990 was married with two children, despite previously being told she might never be able to have them.

When asked to comment at the time, Stephen said he had an 85 per cent success rate:

> Before I saw [Lynne] I meditated on her case. When I first met her I felt I could help. I asked for the power and it came. Sometimes when I am laying on my hands, they get very hot. I have burned two people by mistake ...
>
> Spiritualist healing has been scientifically proved. I feel I have a gift which I must use for the benefit of other people. Most people come to me when hospitals and doctors can do no more.

The phenomenon of hands-on healing was gaining some early scientific acceptance in the USA at this time. Two years earlier, Dolores (now Professor) Krieger's first study had been published, appearing to demonstrate that Therapeutic Touch, a systematic method of hands-on healing developed for use by nurses in American hospitals, raised haemoglobin levels in volunteers. Later, following further proof, Therapeutic Touch was incorporated into the nursing curriculum in a number of states.

Meanwhile Stephen himself fell ill again, this time with meningitis. Once again, though, after suffering for a relatively short time, he recovered very quickly.

For the next five years, Stephen worked at his job during the day and gave healing late into the evenings after his mediation. Healing exhibitions and demonstrations were performed at the weekends.

The healing path is not the easiest of journeys, however, and can certainly put a strain on a relationship where one partner is not involved as much as the other. Stephen and Jean grew apart during these years and in 1980 decided to separate.

The following year, Stephen met a woman called Kathy, who had also not long been separated. In order to earn some extra money, she had started working in a pub in the evening after a long day at the distribution company where she was a manager. Understandably, her energy levels were very low and had been for some months. She and her mother, Elisabeth, had previously visited a psychic surgeon called George Chapman a number of times whilst he was conducting his surgery in Aylesbury. When he moved to Wales, it was too far to travel, so when Kathy heard about Stephen, she immediately resolved to see him as quickly as possible. But after the first two sessions, there was no change at all in her energy levels.

'I'm sorry, Kathleen,' said Stephen apologetically. 'I just don't understand it. It seems like you are being drained of all the healing I put into you.'

On her next visit Kathy had a surprise waiting for her.

'What are you doing here?' demanded the big man as she walked through the door.

'I'm, I'm here for my appointment,' stuttered Kathy, wondering what had got into the generally jovial Stephen.

'No, not you, YOU!' he shouted, pointing above her left shoulder as he advanced towards her. Scared, Kathy considered a hasty exit.

'Don't worry, Kathleen, I can see the cause of your problems now,' said Stephen in a more comforting tone. 'You've got a leech in your aura. An old man with nothing better to do than hang around pubs and get his fix by latching onto you.'

Stephen held the aura vampire in a mental cage and talked to him, while simultaneously calling for his spirit guide, Chan, who in turn summoned other guides specializing in a certain type of rescue work. Chan asked the old man his name and began explaining to him that he had been unfortunate in not receiving proper guidance on his transition to the spirit world because he had unwittingly chosen a vibration which corresponded with his lower thoughts and therefore had become 'lost' on passing over.

'You see, my friend,' Chan continued, 'there are millions of vibrational states which correspond to the quality of your thought patterns. There are many much more satisfying states than the one you chose on your passing. It is always a good time to move onwards and upwards, but it must be your choice. I cannot determine the rate of your spiritual progress for you. How do you feel about what I have said?'

Face to face with the power of the pure love emanating from the highly evolved beings now surrounding him, the old man began to understand and he smiled a little and asked if they knew how he could find his older brothers and sisters who had passed over many years before him. Chan was visibly delighted as he and the spirit entourage disappeared with their most recent rescuee, leaving Stephen to fill in the gaps for a very bemused patient.

'Basically,' he said, 'a man who had led a life of drinking and debauchery on Earth passed over to the spirit world in that state of mind and, with no guidance from higher beings, he decided it must be quite natural to carry on in the same old way. As he no longer had the physical attributes necessary to enjoy a drink in the same manner as he did on Earth, he had to find a "host" who was depleted enough so that he could invade and exit their energy field, the aura, at will. That host would also have to be taking a drink regularly, so he waited around pubs until he found the right set of circumstances and you were his choice. The first two times you came to see me, he had scarpered before you got here but this time he had become entwined in your energy field and couldn't get out before you arrived.'

Thinking this was all a bit strange, Kathy quickly made her excuses and headed home. But the next day she felt fantastic. She wondered whether there really had been an old spirit man sucking on her energy field. Her son, Mark, had a 'twisted' kidney problem and all conventional avenues had been exhausted. She took him to Stephen.

'Mark said it felt as if someone's hand went inside, grabbed the kidney and wrenched it,' she reports today. 'All I know is that my son got better when all other treatment had got us absolutely nowhere. I began to believe that Stephen really was serious when he spoke of different dimensions and the help that we can get from beings who live on other levels of reality. I went back to him. One thing led to another and we began seeing each other regularly.'

In 1982, Stephen's divorce was granted and Kathy's came through on the same day. A little later, they were married. They moved to 81 West Belvedere in Danbury and Stephen carried on his job and did healing in the evenings, with Kathy helping him.

Then, after three years of this relative tranquillity, their lives took an amazing turn.

4

GROWTH:
THE PSYCHIC SURGEON

There is a principle which is a bar against all
information, which is proof against all argument,
and cannot fail to keep a man in everlasting ignorance. That principle is condemnation before
investigation.

HERBERT SPENCER

It was 1 July 1985 and the day began just like any other for
Stephen. He got up, got ready, went to work and came home
to eat and then prepare for the evening's healing appointments. However, in the late afternoon, Linda, a friend from
Southend, called for urgent help.

By the early evening, when Stephen and Kathy arrived,
she was in a dreadful state. 'Oh thank goodness. My back's
terrible. As you can see I can hardly stand.'

She was obviously in pain. They laid her on the kitchen
table and Stephen began contact healing. As usual the heat
generated by his healing hands soothed Linda's aching back.
Then, just as he was about to finish, 'In 20 minutes, we will
operate!' said a stern Germanic voice in his head. Linda and
Kathy looked perplexed as Stephen appeared to be listening to
someone who wasn't there.

'A very powerful spirit has just told me that we will operate in 20 minutes. I'll have to go into trance. Is that alright
with everybody?'

Linda had known Stephen for some time and trusted him completely. She and Kathy watched as he prepared himself for deep trance. Sitting in a chair, his eyes slowly closed and his head fell forwards until it could fall no further. There his body sat, limp and motionless, except for the occasional deep and heavy breath. After a few minutes, it appeared as though electric shocks were being administered to him. Dr Kahn had begun removing Stephen from his body. Suddenly, the spirit surgeon had taken over.

'I will not be working on your back but on the stomach,' he declared.

'That would make sense,' agreed Linda, 'I've just been to the hospital and the doctor diagnosed an ovarian cyst.'

'That is correct,' said the good doctor. He went on to explain that it was the cyst which was creating the pain in her back, displaying a mastery of medicine that Stephen definitely did not have.

Gesturing for Linda to be helped back on to the table, the austere but kindly doctor used his fingers to mimic the actions of giving an injection. This caused a lump the size of a grape to come up. It immediately began to go a mauve colour and Linda became drowsy. The whole room started to smell of ether, a substance which, they later learned, was used in operating theatres when Dr Kahn was working on Earth.

Stephen sat with his eyes closed, breathing loudly and nasally. 'Dr Kahn appeared to be having some problems controlling Stephen's body,' Kathy told me. 'He kept grumbling under his breath and moving Stephen's head around as if he was looking for something.' (Dr Kahn can 'see' even if Stephen's eyes are closed.) Then Dr Kahn leant back and reached over to the draining board. He casually selected a sharp kitchen knife and Kathy watched in horror as he began to perform an operation on Linda.

With the operation over, Dr Kahn vacated Stephen's body in much the same way as he had entered it. As Stephen opened his eyes, Linda was rolling around on the table, groaning and holding her stomach. This turned out to be due to shock and delayed nervousness rather than any real discomfort.

'How do you feel?' asked Kathy.

'The pain in my back has gone,' replied Linda.

A subsequent visit to the hospital confirmed that the growth had gone too.

This then, was the start of one of the most successful partnerships in psychic surgery – on a kitchen table in Southend-on-Sea!

The operations continued. In 1986 Stephen began working on Saturday afternoons at Dr Billie Mansfield's house in Cranbrook Road, Ilford. At that time, he was performing, on average, 10 operations per session.

In these early days Stephen would have to sit down in a chair for most of the time and Kathy would help him move around the table, assisting by handing the instruments when Dr Kahn requested them. Stephen's eyes were always closed at first, until the spirit team found a way to open them. But to begin with Stephen just stared piercingly, without blinking at all. This was somewhat frightening for the patients as well as being bad for Stephen.

It was in this early period that Mr James was first mentioned by Dr Kahn. One day, Kathy was standing next to Stephen, who was sitting on a stool at the head of the prone patient.

'Pass me the spike,' ordered Dr Kahn. 'I am going to do a frontal lobotomy.' Kathy reached for 'the spike' but, before she could even get to it, a hole began appearing in the middle of the patient's forehead.

'You must be quicker, Katerina,' smiled Dr Kahn. 'Mr James is working very quickly today. You must try to keep up, my dear.'

In the early days, the Turoffs asked many questions of and about the spirit team but were generally told that information would be forthcoming on a 'need to know' basis. Both Stephen and Kathy have long since decided that, as long as the healing is helping people, trying to discover all the details is an irrelevant and time-wasting exercise. Perhaps more information will become available in the future.

About a year after Mr James was first introduced, Stephen's eyes were open but still not blinking. This made them very sore, but then the spirit team managed to get them to blink and to activate the tear ducts so that he could be in deep trance for up to eight hours per day. Nowadays, the technique has advanced so much that light trance control is sufficient; Stephen is fully conscious and any one or more of 18 members of the spirit team come in and out of his energy field at will, depending on the patient's requirements. One of the reasons for this development is the sheer number of people being treated. Another is that Stephen's own spiritual progress would not be furthered if he continued to vacate his body during the healing work.

Throughout the early part of 1987, the strain of working as a carpenter during the day and performing deep trance healing each evening was beginning to tell on Stephen's health. In prayers one night he asked for guidance and a fortnight later was unexpectedly made redundant. This forced him to consider healing on a full-time basis. Two weeks later he had earned a grand total of £10 and was wondering what on Earth had made him even consider trying to make a living from his healing gift!

Still he persevered and later that same year had a breakthrough when he was offered the use of treatment rooms at the Barbican, London, on Thursdays. This came about through an acquaintance called Mitzy who had been impressed by Stephen's healing and had a friend, an American doctor called Linda Chard, who had the rooms. Dr Chard kept detailed records of the psychic surgery and later published a number of case histories in her book, *Dr Kahn: The Spirit Surgeon* (Elmore-Chard, 1992). She studied the psychic surgery phenomenon at close hand for nearly five years and concluded:

> *We know that Stephen is not masquerading. He is taken over by a being, identified as Dr Joseph Kahn from the Spirit World, who performs psychic surgery with physical instruments powered by energies of a type which are still unknown to man ... I have seen a doctor, dead to the earth plane, perform operations that defy normal scientific interpretation.*
>
> *When I first met Stephen, I had no personal experience of psychic surgery ... Now, after more than four years, I realize that my 'educated' mind still blinkers my vision and inhibits a full understanding of what takes place ...*
>
> *My understanding of what Dr Kahn does when de-materializing diseased tissue is that by altering the sub-atomic energy within the cellular structure of the tissue he is able to disperse it into recyclable matter. The reader may believe that 'de-materialization' is something straight from science fiction; but whatever its reality, it has been part of the cure for many of our patients.*
>
> *The reverse of de-materialization is 'materialization'. This we have also seen in our clinic.*

Stephen and the spirit team were achieving such consistently good results that the media began to take a serious interest in the Danbury and Barbican clinics. In the summer of 1988, in its 25 June issue, *Psychic News* published some of the independently received testimonies of patients who had been to see Stephen and Dr Kahn. The article was entitled: 'Healer's hand penetrates bodies as far as knuckles – say patients' and began:

> An entranced British healer's hand 'appeared to disappear as far as the knuckles right into the patient's body through her back'. This is just one of the astounding testimonies received on the latest development in the work of Stephen Turoff. Two patients, independently, told PN: 'It seemed as though his hand was right in my stomach.' Another testified she saw the spirit doctor's hand pass 'through the flesh and into my body'. 'Injections' were felt by the patients, and many spoke of sensing something cold being 'poured' into them.

Stephen told the newspaper that once he had asked his guide if he could watch the spirit surgery:

> I could see everything happening in my head – in colour. That really put me off! Once we used some water and a little blood materialized in it. I don't like blood and asked Dr Kahn to stop that. Now patients say they are getting a sticky feeling around where the operation takes place. Scars come; and go within about three days.

Because of the unique form the healing was apparently taking, *Psychic News* asked for handwritten testimonials from patients who had experienced it. Among those who responded were some who had undergone treatment from the spirit surgeon a while before. T. M. Watt of Basildon, Essex, sent a letter certifying that he had accompanied a patient and witnessed two psychic operations:

> The first one was to remove a blood clot from Dot Keefe's left breast, this being done through her clothing. She was given an injection, which she did not feel, and Dr Kahn appeared to cut open her chest. After he had removed the clot, he said he was going to pour something into her that might feel cold.
>
> In the second spirit operation, Dot did feel the injection, and a mark like a pinprick remained on her arm. The spirit doctor operated on the bare flesh for lower back pain. This time he made no move to cut her, but, with a circular movement of his fingers, his hand appeared to disappear as far as the knuckles right into her body through her back.
>
> [Dot asked Mr Watt to look at her back the following day.] Two scars could clearly be seen and they lasted for approximately one week.

Writing to thank Stephen, the patient gave a glowing testimony:

> I am now completely free of back pain. I felt the injection in my arm. When Dr Kahn said he was going to pour something into my back that may feel cold it certainly was.

S. N. Burley of Chelmsford also wrote to tell of his experiences:

> I have had several spirit operations from Dr Kahn, all of which had been performed on the etheric body, but this last encounter was quite different. Dr Kahn informed me that he now operated entirely on the

physical body. [The injection] wasn't actually painful, but one knew that a needle had been inserted.

[The spirit surgeon had warned him that the operation would cause some discomfort.] This was quite true. At times it was almost unbearable, but some of the pain could have been due to fear as I realized what Dr Kahn was doing. After the incision, which was painless, his hand appeared to penetrate right through my flesh and muscle. It seemed as though his hand was right in my stomach. He twisted and probed, and then poured some plasma into the area, which he said would be cold – and it was.

The operation lasted for at least 10 minutes. When I dismounted from the couch I felt really weak and sore. I had expected to feel worse, but several hours later when the effect of the anaesthetic had worn off, I really was in pain. The scar was very pronounced and my flesh was red and bruised.

According to Mr Burley, for three days the pain was 'very bad, but it gradually eased a little'. Then, writing four days after the spirit operation, he stated, 'I am feeling much better,' and ended his letter:

This must be a new dimension in spiritual healing, and I feel highly honoured to know that I am one of the first people to experience such a unique physical operation.

Hilda Ferris of Danbury Common also testified to witnessing Dr Kahn's 'operative hand passed through the flesh and into my body. He then proceeded to remove something fibrous from my pancreas.' She attested, 'Never have I experienced this kind of physical manipulation for operations before.'

J. Cullen of Gidea Park told Stephen: 'It felt as if Dr Kahn's hand was right inside my stomach. In fact the friend who accompanied me said during the operation she could not see most of his hand, which appeared to have penetrated right inside me.'

In 1988, Karen Menzies of the London *Evening Standard* came to Stephen to be treated for a whiplash injury and the story of her experience appeared in the Monday 27 June issue under the heading, 'The doctor is way out – this healer's bedside manner comes straight from the twilight zone'. The article was written in a slightly sensationalist style, but it was obvious that the journalist had had an interesting experience, to say the least:

> *The XR3 fraternity would doubtless describe 40-year-old Stephen Turoff as 'a good bloke'. A strapping Cockney fellow and a carpenter by trade, he lives in suburban neatness in Chelmsford, enjoys a pint and makes a mean cup of tea. He's a laugh is Stephen. Immensely likeable, down to earth, a little dyslexic, but by no means stupid, and certainly not a chap you'd expect to know a whole lot about ovarian cysts. Nor would you imagine him to suddenly go into trance, assume a (very convincing) German accent and perform psychic operations. But Stephen's a dab hand at all three. He's a channeller, through whom the spirits can make contact with we mere mortals.*

It was shortly after this that I met Stephen and became fascinated by his work and his way of life. I am not alone. Many, many people have been inspired by Stephen's work and words. He explains it like this:

If God had decided to take some positive affirmative action on Earth in order to get things back on track and wanted to attract the attention of any soul who was prepared to help, what better way than creating a centre of intensity which would draw prospective helpers like a magnet? Those who come and go away thinking they have had something less than a spiritual experience are freely able to choose that response. For those souls who are attracted to our work, there is an opportunity to find out more and a choice whether to contribute their time and effort to whatever task God then sets for them.

In my own case, I almost immediately began taking carload upon carload of people over to the clinic for healing. After about four years of this, I asked Stephen why I seemed to be so drawn to the whole thing. He just said, 'You could probably be quite a good healer. Perhaps you should have a go.' Of course, straightaway I set about putting my hands on anyone who would let me and my head swelled as one or two reported feeling a little better afterwards. But over time I learned that each of us has different skills and attributes, and God has given us the gifts of free will and self-determination in order that we can choose how to use our various talents. My own talents might be best put towards promoting the work rather than becoming a psychic surgeon myself, as was my original hope.

All this talk of psychic surgery, spiritual experiences and so on is often a bit much to take in at first. But I can only explain it as it appears to me and countless others. This is the way it is. And why shouldn't there be things that we haven't had knowledge and experience of? Once we start asking serious questions, perhaps we should brace ourselves for some surprising answers.

Early in 1989, husband and wife George and Joan came to see Stephen from Reading. They were pleased with the healing and recommended friends who lived in Fuengirola, Spain. Esteban Molina was an estate and travel agent and had organized venues for Spiritualist meetings in the Malaga region. George and Joan made an appointment for him and his English wife Eileen to come over to Danbury in February 1989. Eileen had knee problems. Esteban asked Dr Kahn, 'Would you be interested in a trip to Spain?'

Dr Kahn smiled at Kathy. Just a few days earlier he had told her, 'Keep your bags packed and your passport up-to-date. My medium will be working abroad in eight months.'

Esteban went back to Spain to make the arrangements and organize the advertising. He was able to generate a large amount of interest in the trip.

In the meantime, Stephen was featured on a BBC Radio programme called *Under the Christian Carpet*, a series in which interviewers George and Trish Target visit small churches that receive little publicity. Stephen was the guest medium for a church in the heart of Norwich and was described as 'an interesting mixture of a man, one minute coming on strong, like a stand-up comedian, telling jokes and making us laugh, and the next, serious, talking of spiritual things... Though he obviously couldn't bring everybody a message of comfort, he'd do his best for as many as possible.'

On Wednesday 4 October 1989, exactly eight months after Dr Kahn had first predicted it, Stephen was doing his best in Spain. He and Kathy were guests of the Spiritual Association of Andalusia. There were healing sessions, lectures and demonstrations of psychic phenomena. Swabs were handed over to patients for further medical examination and analysis.

Halfway through the trip, Dr Kahn suddenly looked up from the operating table, said, 'I need something sharper!' and sent Kathy out to the shops for the sharpest penknife she could find. The letter-opener he had been using was too blunt for the number of people being seen and the speed with which he had to perform the operations if he was to get them done in the time allotted. The hours were difficult – 9 a.m.–2 p.m. in trance, then siesta, then 4.30 p.m.–8.00 p.m. in trance again. This was physically very difficult to accomplish and Stephen was exhausted after each session.

Evidence of Dr Kahn's medical expertise was apparent when he treated a local reflexologist for a problem that the patient was aware of but had not told anyone about. Mike Churchill, of Benalmadena Pueblo, was seeking help for a painful wrist, but the healer began treating his chest and one of his kidneys. Mr Churchill confessed he suffered badly with asthma – 'It caused extreme discomfort every morning when I woke up' – and was treated in front of 300 wide-eyed witnesses.

'The doctor told me he had inserted a tube into my lung,' he added. 'And it's absolutely marvellous now. I have no asthma at all.' The operation involved large incisions in the patient's chest and side and lasted about five minutes in all. Later, when friends suggested that he must have imagined it, he showed them the scar. Operation scars are difficult to explain away as imagination!

That same month, in an interview with *Psychic News*, which was published under the heading 'UK healer "operates" in Spain', Señor Molina explained the purpose of the visit:

During the past year the Spanish association's main aim has been to raise enough funds for a spiritual centre. We live in a country where it is very difficult to promote Spiritualism. It will take a lot of effort to bring things up to the standard that many Spiritualists take for granted in the United Kingdom. The country needs Spiritualist churches and more healers and clairvoyants ... We need all the help we can

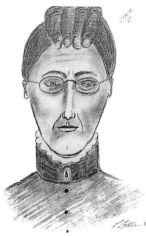

Left This is a sketch drawing by psychic artist Len Lobban. The artist 'saw' Grace standing beside Elsebe, a South African friend of Stephen's, when she commissioned him to do a portrait.
© *Len Lobban*

Below This is the photograph of Nurse Grace which Stephen found at a hospital in east London, many months *after* the sketch drawing was sent to him by Elsebe.

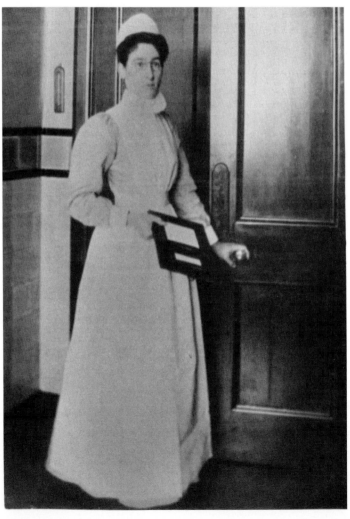

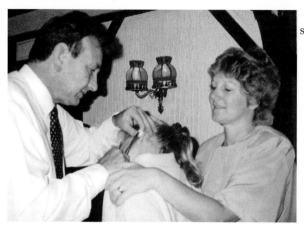

Right Knives, scalpels, scissors, water, flannels, cotton wool and vibhuti (sacred ash) are the simple tools of the psychic surgeon.
© *Tim Cavanagh*

Above Stephen and his wife Kathy work together in their front room which became a makeshift 'operating theatre' in the early days of the psychic surgery.

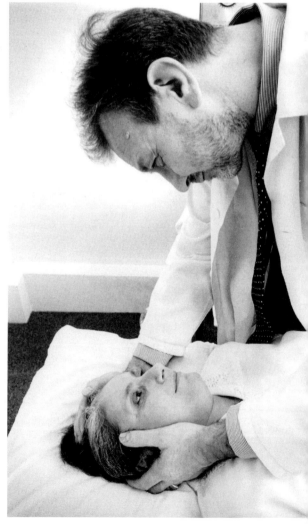

Right Stephen often stares into a patient's eyes, transfixing them for minutes at a time, before offering some words of encouragement or advice.

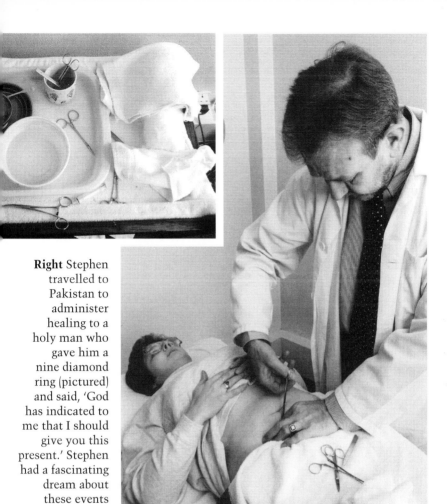

Right Stephen travelled to Pakistan to administer healing to a holy man who gave him a nine diamond ring (pictured) and said, 'God has indicated to me that I should give you this present.' Stephen had a fascinating dream about these events beforehand.

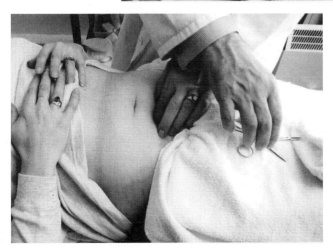

Left Patients often report feeling a sensation of being cut open and of hands and instruments moving about inside them. Scars generally heal within a few days.

© *Tim Cavanagh*

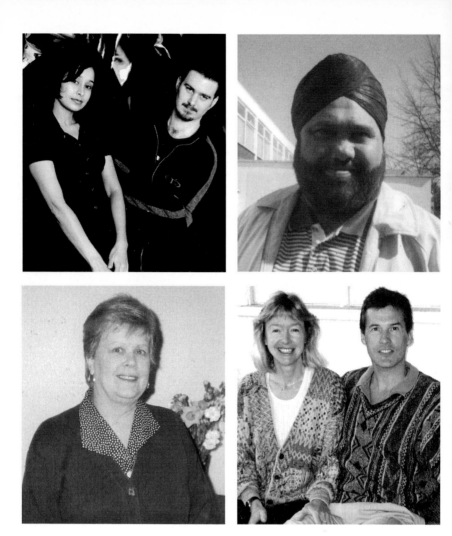

Top left Sonya Madan is singer and lyricist with the rock group Echobelly. She will never forget her experience of psychic surgery: 'I'm very grateful to Stephen Turoff for helping me.'
© *Ray Burmiston*

Top right Originally from Uganda, Mr Khamba went to Stephen with swollen arthritic knees and chest pains. After one visit he reported: 'The swelling in my knees has completely gone and my chest pain has eased considerably.'
© *Jane Solomon*

Above left Ann Bradford is a childminder who went to Stephen with breast cancer. She said, 'I remember thinking, Ow! He's cut me, but it didn't hurt. It was as if I had been given a local anaesthetic ... All I could think about was the mess the blood would make on my white jumper.'
© *Sarah Bradford*

Above right Dr Tim Ewer and his partner Julie Searle visited Stephen to conduct research and experience psychic surgery at first hand.

get. The association is now hoping to move to a permanent centre. Stephen's visit raised about 350,000 pesetas which will be put towards a new centre.

Meanwhile, interest in Stephen's work at home was gradually increasing. At the end of 1989, an article by journalist Charles Yates of the *Sport* newspaper appeared alongside photographs of the Nurse Grace psychic drawing, a patient cured of a perforated eardrum and Stephen/Dr Kahn performing 'invisible surgery'. Whilst this article was inevitably tabloid in its approach and written ever-so-slightly 'tongue in cheek', it brought up a rather interesting point about the 'latest private threat to Britain's NHS'. Stephen and Dr Kahn would not want to be a threat to any person or any organization, but Dr Kahn is on video, at Dr Linda Chard's clinic, predicting that this form of spirit/human medical co-operation will expand greatly in the future and provide a whole new way of looking at the diagnosis and treatment of dis-ease. Apparently, it is as much a question of the spirit world learning to lower their vibrations and get the science right on their side as it is of us on Earth learning to raise our vibrations and get all the conditions right on our side. When the time is right, predicts Dr Kahn, this new form of 'holistic', cheap medicine, which dispenses with anaesthetics and powerful drugs, together with their unwanted side-effects, will usher in a new era of medical techniques.

Despite their healing success, the nineties began for the Tur-off family with continuing financial troubles. For some time Kathy and Stephen had been worried about their circumstances; they were seeing a lot of people, but many for no charge and others for very little. In conversation with Dr Kahn, Kathy had mentioned their concerns and he had told her not to worry as she would be getting 'a rather nice birthday present'. She could not understand this as they barely had enough for essentials, let alone lavish presents!

The present actually arrived the day after Kathy's birthday. A *News of the World* reporter, Trevor Kempson, who had called and requested healing, contributed to an article entitled: 'The carpenter who cures sick with a penknife', which appeared on Sunday 7 January 1990. The article was so supportive of their healing work that thousands of people wanted to know more.

'The phone didn't stop ringing,' says Kathy. 'The local telephone exchange actually gave up, due to the volume of calls which got diverted all over the area. The mail was delivered in huge post office sacks. It was certainly a surprise present from Dr Kahn and the spirit healing team – but we've come to expect the unexpected from them nowadays.'

Eleven days later the Turoffs were off to Fuengirola on their second visit to Spain. While they were there, *Psychic News*, in their 20 January issue, reported the excitement caused by the *News of the World* article earlier in the month. Once again, 'the phone didn't stop when we arrived home'.

News of Stephen's miraculous cures spread still more widely. In April the Turoffs set off on a third trip to Spain and in June they travelled to Sweden as guests of the Swedish Spiritualist Association. This trip included a demonstration of transfiguration, in which images of the 'dead' and 'deities' appear on Stephen's face, often in front of large audiences. He has done this many times for such diverse individuals and groups of people as a criminal psychologist, a Bishop who witnessed the room 'lighting up and Jesus appearing on Stephen's face' and Hindu, Moslem and other religious leaders who tell of visions relating to their own traditions. Numerous other testimonies tell of the appearance of sundry relatives and spirit guides. I have personally witnessed this incredible phenomenon and watching a transfiguration can only be described as a moving experience.

Stephen was entranced in front of the 43 Spiritualists in the church. His Chinese guide, Chan, spoke to them in broken English. Several loved ones of the congregation members were brought through to superimpose their features on the medium's face.

'One was a boy in his twenties who had "died" in a car crash,' explained Stephen. 'His head was crushed. He had a hole in it. When he transfigured me, he showed the hole in his head with blood running from it.'

Other spirit communicators came through and held conversations with the audience in Swedish. Stephen doesn't speak a word of that language!

Later on, Chan returned to explain that there were many 'spirit children' present. 'If you keep quiet,' he added, 'you will hear them.' A hush spread over the congregation and they were able to hear children's voices. Next Chan asked for a small table to be brought to the cabinet where Stephen sat. He asked Kathy to get up and place her hands on the table and also for one of the audience to come up and touch the table. It moved up and down, danced, and did all sorts of different things for the entertainment of the audience.

The demonstration of transfiguration then continued. A woman manifested who said she was Helen Duncan. Helen was one of Britain's most outstanding and respected 'physical' mediums. She was arrested and convicted under the Fraudulent Mediums Act during World War II because servicemen killed in action communicated at her séances – before news of their passing had been publicly released. Both Kathy and the church president's wife were familiar with books on the medium, and testified they recognized her face. Helen said she was going to show some of her work. Ectoplasm came out of Stephen's mouth and lay on his chest. It was not dense, more like a white cloud. This stayed for two or three minutes then seemed to be sucked back into his mouth. The communicating entity spoke for a couple of minutes to the audience, then left the medium. Stephen was later told that the entity had spoken in a Scottish accent, just like Mrs Duncan. He said, 'I am not a physical medium as such, so these phenomena were all a bit new to me.'

Stephen was, however, delighted with Kathy's rapidly developing mediumship and Dr Kahn urged Kathy to sit for development, mentioning that prescriptions would be transmitted. 'I had a job to get her to sit,' Stephen said. Yet the first time Kathy did sit, back in Britain, the table moved immediately. Though not levitating, it started darting all over the place. This happens not only in darkness, but also in broad daylight. Kathy's power was growing. She started receiving prescriptions. Though in automatic writing, they resembled ordinary handwritten notes, not with the words linked up as normally occurs. Kathy's eyes were closed and her head averted as her hand moved across the paper. The writing came thick and furiously. Stephen was delighted, seeing this as an adjunct to his healing mission. Some Swedish patients had the prescriptions made up and many were found to be homoeopathic. The script was completely different from Kathy's and messages from recipients' loved ones were in their own handwriting. Their accuracy of content was vouched for in every case.

When Dr Kahn performed spirit operations in Sweden, assisted by the church president and his wife, large blood clots were seen, photographed and taken away. Several measured 3 inches (8 cm) across. Dr Kahn thrust a 6-inch knife into a male patient's nose to withdraw one large clot. A heart sufferer had a metal object pushed into his chest and blood clots materialized with the incision.

'The body closed within minutes,' said Stephen. 'Dr Kahn just puts his hand over the incision and it closes.'

News of the happenings soon spread around Sweden. 'The press just hounded me,' Stephen said. Though invited on TV, he declined. 'I was told I would be locked up, because I am using knives.'

Back home, Kathy's table-moving continued and has developed into occasional table-dancing with a 'Mr MacPherson', who tells us that he died in a major Scottish battle hundreds of years ago. Stephen simply puts on Mr MacPherson's favourite Highland jig and within seconds he is there. I have seen him materialize on Stephen's face during transfiguration. He has a great big mop of hair and a huge bushy beard. Kathy charges the table and off it goes around the room. For those of you who hold that seeing is believing, this one is worth a look!

Precisely because metaphysical and paranormal phenomena are difficult to accept without first-hand experience, Stephen and Kathy were travelling to many venues at the weekends to demonstrate the psychic surgery. One Saturday, 13 July 1990, turned out to be very unlucky for a man who obviously had trouble accepting what he was seeing with his own eyes.

Stephen and Kathy had arrived at Toftwood Hall, East Dereham, Norfolk, with time to spare and had set up the operating table and all the instruments at the front of the hall. All went well initially until a very regrettable thing happened. A young man, obviously sceptical, ran from the back of the hall, snatched a blood clot that had been removed from the lung of one of the patients and which was now being passed around for inspection, and popped it into his mouth in some sort of protest that it was all a show. He had not, presumably, been present when Stephen had explained, as usual, that all tissue removed from patients could be taken away to be analysed by any doctor or laboratory as long as a small sample remained with the Turoffs to prevent switching and misrepresentation.

'You stupid boy!' exclaimed Dr Kahn. 'That tissue is diseased and you have swallowed it. Get to your doctor as soon as possible and tell him what you have done.'

Needless to say, the protester became a bit more convinced and hurriedly left the hall. As far as is known, however, nothing serious subsequently happened to him.

When one lady did take blood removed by Dr Kahn to her own doctor, the GP sent it away to be analysed. The patient was then summoned back to see the very bemused physician.

'Where did you get this blood from?'

'It was taken from my body during psychic surgery.'

'But, that's impossible. It's literally full of cancer!'

'Well, that's what happened,' the lady insisted. The doctor promised to look into the matter, but nothing seems to have ever come of it.

This sums up the response of many doctors. Initially they are shocked and go through a denial process. When they witness psychic surgery for themselves or cannot get the patient to change the story, they tend to just leave it at that and get on with practising what they know – orthodox, Western allopathic medicine. A few try to compare the spiritually inspired techniques used by Dr Kahn with the practice of modern medicine. But this is like comparing 'trepanning' – skull-drilling as practised by primitive people circa 4000 BC – with modern brain surgery. Both are apparently an operation performed in the area of the head but they are very different, and therefore not comparable, in many important ways.

A modern doctor tends to see patients as physical machines with broken parts. The purpose of the medicine is to isolate, label and then attack the symptom with drugs, radiation or surgery. The underlying cause of the 'dis-ease' is often relegated to second place on the scale of importance.

By contrast, Dr Kahn has learned to see patients as a swirling, vibrating, kaleidoscopic mass of sub-atomic energy which incorporates, and is the vehicle of expression for, the 'primary cosmic travelling atom', the individual consciousness. He can read your Akashic record, the 'videotape' of everything you have ever done in this life and before, which gives him an indication of where the current conditions you have created for yourself are likely to lead you in the next few years of this present Earth life experience. His medicine works on the levels of your mental, spiritual and emotional as well as physical self. He uses otherworldly knowledge of biology, chemistry and physics in order to balance and harmonize your 'whole', which may be in a state of disequilibrium through the conditions which you have created for yourself (or which may have been created for you) as part of your case-book of character-building experiences.

A consultation with this highly evolved and benevolent being can lead to an advance for your soul which would otherwise take many lifetimes to achieve. He can help you create conditions for yourself in which the path you were on can be altered to your eternal benefit and that of the single universal consciousness.

It is, we are told, *never* an accident or coincidence that you find yourself in consultation with Dr Kahn. Whether or not the experience appears to be good or bad at the time is irrelevant. You were meant to be there and you received what you needed for your inexorable progress Home ... to your Divine Mother and Father, to God.

By the middle of July 1990 the demands for healing had reached such proportions that Kathy had been forced to give up her job as a distribution company manager in order to concentrate on helping Stephen with the healing clinic. No rest for the good or the wicked, it seems!

On 6 August, Stephen and Kathy took up an invitation to be filmed during a demonstration at Pitsea, Basildon. One of

Kathy's former colleagues at the distribution company, Simon Eakins, was 'curious' to capture events with his own video camera.

The resulting video is a very graphic example of psychic surgery actually being performed in front of an audience. In one operation, the finger of the surgeon quite clearly goes into an eye socket about an inch deep, with no discomfort reported by the patient. One remarkable aspect of this video is that, although Dr Kahn and the team allowed everything else to be shown, it appears that they paranormally edited out one part of an operation. This was a section in which a woman who had suffered from terrible headaches for many years submitted to having a 6-inch (15 cm) letter-opener inserted up her nasal passage and twisted to release a 'massive blood clot' which she then spat out into a kidney bowl when she sat up in front of the large audience of witnesses. Everybody saw what happened. The lady was even given the diseased tissue to take home.

This certainly helped to persuade Simon Eakins of the awesome power at the disposal of the spirit team. But this and many other similar events surrounding the 'Turoff phenomenon' pose more questions than they offer answers. Perhaps that is the point. Perhaps God is increasing our exposure to things we cannot explain in order to 'open our minds' for what is soon to come?

In November 1990, *Psychic News* once again covered the Turoffs' latest visit to the Costa del Sol and the trip was also reported in a six-page illustrated feature in *Pronto*, Spain's biggest selling magazine, and a double-page spread in *El Sol*, which is circulated in southern Spain. Two Canary Island newspapers also published accounts. Stephen told reporters, 'Sometimes I feel scared about this gift. It has got more and more physical. But Dr Kahn does it because he says, "Seeing is believing. In your world today they need to see." '

One of the Spanish newspapers sent two journalists who were so impressed with what they saw that they returned with a cameraman asking permission to take close-up photographs. Stephen, as usual, agreed. Several photographs were printed, including one showing the 4-inch (10-cm) blades of a pair of scissors disappearing into the nostrils of a patient.

'Sometimes,' said Stephen, 'Dr Kahn takes clots out of patients' bodies. A kidney bowl is filled with blood and lumps. At other times, he wraps gauze around a pair of scissors and pushes them right up into the nostrils. Or, he might make a cut directly into the body and people see blood flow. He has often used a spike to draw out blood clots which are black and lumpy. These things are accepted far more readily in some foreign countries than in Britain.'

The Turoffs ended their interviews by telling of the new Dr Joseph Kahn Healing Centre which had been set up near Fuengirola and their long-term plans to provide accommodation for patients who have travelled some distance. One day, they concluded, they hoped to set up an orphanage alongside the healing centre.

Stephen was then televised at work for the ITV programme *First Tuesday*. 'After seeing the operations, they scrapped it,' he commented. 'It looked too way out.'

At this time, almost in direct proportion to Stephen's success, there seemed to be an increase in the amount of animosity towards him from other mediums and healers. Stephen couldn't understand it. 'We all work for the same Gov'nor to propagate what we believe in, that there is survival after death,' he commented to a journalist, 'so I don't see why people have to have a go at me for proving it day in and day out.'

Also in 1990 there was a new departure for Dr Kahn. He decided that the surgical techniques had advanced sufficiently for a public demonstration of opening the body without using instruments. We are told that the spirit team are working very hard to develop their skills. It is, apparently, time for the Earth plane to be blessed with the early beginnings of medical co-operation with spirit entities. But that means that the spirit people also have to work hard to get it right as part of their own development. Each of the spirit team is still developing as an individual, just as we all are.

The unlikely venue for the first of these operations without instruments was a little place called Peacham Hall in Chingford, London E4. *Psychic News*, as ever, covered the story under the heading ' "Dead" doctor removes cyst during his demonstration':

> *For the first time ever, spirit surgeon Dr Kahn ... demonstrated before a witness his technique of opening up the body without using instruments.*
>
> *... Sandra Coombs ... had been consulting a doctor for the last year because of a cyst in her right cheek. Dr Kahn ran my finger across her face, whereupon a small opening appeared. The cyst was completely removed. When the operation was over, all that remained was a slight blemish. Pieces of foreign matter were carefully collected in a glass and the patient walked away a very happy woman. At no time during the operation did she feel any pain.*

I was at this event and the patient treated was two seats away. When she came back to her place she was beaming. The pus from the cyst had stunk horribly and was offered to the patient to take away in a small jar. Other psychics were asked what they could see as Dr Kahn worked and they reported various colours to the whole audience. People at the front were given the opportunity to request their favourite natural perfume.

'Jasmine, please,' asked one lady.

'Certainly,' said Dr Kahn. Within seconds the water he had rubbed onto his hands became jasmine scented.

It should be mentioned here that, depending on the mindset of the observer, what is seen during psychic surgery can appear completely different to two people at the same event. This can unfortunately give rise to some confusion.

On Valentine's Day 1991, Stephen and Kathy travelled to Mexico for the first time. They had met a Spanish woman – we shall call her 'Sallie' – in 1990, on one of their trips to Spain. Sallie had then brought people from Mexico to the UK for healing and psychic surgery. The Spanish flat she was staying in was owned by a rich Mexican who was very ill and was one of the people that Sallie invited to England to receive healing from Stephen. She turned up again on the next Spanish trip and asked if Stephen would go to Mexico to work. Stephen agreed straightaway. Sallie made all the arrangements and a short while later the Turoffs found themselves arriving in Mexico, complete with winter coats, jumpers, warm undies and footwear, in the middle of a South American heatwave!

Sallie was all smiles at the airport. But the sixth sense of the master psychic started alarm bells ringing and events were to prove him very right. It transpired that Sallie had turned up two months earlier and had very kindly started to take large amounts of money for appointments on Stephen's behalf! Stephen learned that the Mexican organizer of his trip was upset with her for many reasons and, in turn, with Stephen because Sallie was his 'representative'. Stephen normally makes very sure that no one represents him without specific sanction, but he resolved to work on, under a cloud, for the first week until he could sort the whole thing out with the organizers.

He soon found that they were looking forward to meeting him for the very same purpose. He was shown into a huge study which was 'more like that library in *The Godfather*' and the door was slammed shut behind him. Now, the Brick Lane carpenter is a very big man. But the two men in thousand-dollar suits and dark glasses who stood blocking the exit with arms folded, were very, very big men. Hmmm, they're a bit more formal than I remembered, thought Stephen, wondering how far the drop was through the open window.

Suddenly a brown bag landed on the big desk between him and a very red-faced, silver-haired Mexican who was clearly upset about something.

'Why did you prescribe these pills?' the man bellowed. 'Sallie told us you said we had to have these and charged us $7,000 for them.'

Another bag hit the desk.

'And she charged us even more for these for my boy!'

The 'miracle pills' had been tested and shown to be sugar. Many people had been cheated. Even worse, the boy was very sick and had been given false hope by Sallie's cure-all tales. At heart, the wealthy Mexican gentleman was a reasonable man, but this sequence of events would test anyone's patience.

In the end the problem was resolved when Stephen suggested they contact Esteban Molina in Spain. He vouched for Stephen's honesty and the atmosphere lightened. The two large librarians glanced at each other, smiled and unfolded their arms. The Mexican gentleman offered his hand.

With that small hiccough over with, the trip went on to be very enjoyable. Kathy and Stephen spent two very pleasant days in Mexico City as honoured guests of their Latin American hosts. They were treated to the very best of clubs and restaurants, and a special outing to see the ancient pyramids 'provided the icing on the cake and rounded off a wonderful experience very nicely'.

Healing sessions were conducted in the diplomatic suite of the Impala Hotel, Tampico. Over 200 patients were treated by Dr Kahn, including two Roman Catholic priests and a chief of police. The Mexican hosts said that all the patients were completely satisfied. Stephen commented that the amount of people who visited him in Mexico and the reaction he received was 'incredible'.

Stephen was busy at home too. People were travelling from all over the UK to receive healing. Nancy Haigh, a well known Yorkshire clairvoyant and a qualified aromatherapist, told how she saw the entranced Stephen remove an 'enormous clot' from her husband's back:

> He picked up a scalpel and made an incision at the base of Peter's spine. I saw the blood starting to come out. Stephen's wife, Kathy, then lit something, placed it over the incision and put a glass on top of it. This was apparently to draw the clot to the surface. A small towel was placed over the glass. Kathy kept her hands on the towel at each side of it.
>
> When Dr Kahn picked up the cloth later, the glass was three-quarters full of blood. There was an enormous clot inside it. He then told Peter, 'This will heal up.'

Kathy was using a technique known as 'charged cupping'. She was required to 'charge' a glass in order to draw the blood clot to the surface of the body. She would concentrate on sending a positive charge down her right arm, with the left acting as the negative pole. A tingling would occur in the nape of her neck then travel on down her right arm, ending up flowing through the right palm energy centre, causing the hand to rapidly vibrate on the towel placed over the surface of the glass.

The energy created assists the drawing process in some way but Kathy is not sure of the exact mechanism by which it works. Dr Kahn says it is a bit too early for an explanation but we will one day see that this perfectly natural and scientific skill, like all the other techniques used in the psychic surgery, is breathtakingly simple in essence. Perhaps one day we will understand enough about matter, energy, space, time and the other dimensions of reality to make current scientific understanding seem Neanderthal by comparison. And, given the evidence pointing towards the existence of other-dimensional beings, might it not make sense to devote resources to finding a way to contact them in order to help our understanding? How much damage might we avoid by this simple short cut to the truth as opposed to the long, laborious and arduous so-called 'scientific' method that Western science has come to favour?

One scientist, Harry Oldfield, has already devised instruments with which we may be able to communicate with beings from other dimensions. This metaphysical aspect of his work is an interesting, if wholly unintentional, potential use for his inventions, which were designed for medical research. For more on Harry's work, *see* pp.130–5.

In April 1991, Stephen and Kathy were again in Spain, at the invitation of the World Congress of Natural Medicines. At one demonstration over 60 doctors witnessed Dr Kahn turn water into oil to treat a patient. The instruments were laid out on a table for inspection by three of the doctors. A bowl of water was also called for, placed upon the table and examined. Stephen's first patient was a man in his fifties who had suffered from a heart attack.

'He was asked to remove his shirt and lie upon the healing couch,' Stephen explained. 'I was then taken over by Dr

Kahn, who asked one of the doctors to come up from the audience. Dr Kahn handed him the palms of my hands to prove there was nothing on them. He also proved that the water had not been tampered with. Dr Kahn placed one of my hands into the water, withdrew it and rubbed the water onto the patient's chest. It turned immediately into oil.'

The doctor acting as a witness examined the oil. Others were summoned from the audience to confirm there was no trickery. At the end of the man's treatment there were over 10 doctors standing around the couch.

Two women doctors had water placed between their hands by the spirit surgeon. Asked to think of the perfume they wished for while they rubbed their hands, they discovered that it materialized after three minutes.

The next patient was a man who had a back problem. He undressed and laid face down on the couch. Dr Kahn placed a white towel over the lower part of his back and told the doctors he would solidify the healing colour so that it would be seen. They all testified to witnessing a pink light emanating from the palms of Stephen's hands. The spirit doctor removed a blood clot from the base of the patient's back, which was studied by the doctors. Afterwards the patient was able to touch his toes with 'no pain' and was 'very happy'.

With another back sufferer, water was again rubbed into the patient, a woman, but this time with different results. Dr Kahn said he was materializing 'calcified bone and some poison'. The water upon the woman's back could be seen to turn a brown colour with small white particles in it. It was spooned off and examined by a doctor while the patient got up, able to move freely.

This attendance at the World Congress of Natural Medicines opened a number of doors for the Turoffs. Their foreign trips continued, including one to Portugal in which over 170 people were treated, and a video was made of Dr Kahn doing an operation in which his finger enters an eye socket to the depth of about an inch. He looks up and says, 'Do not try this at home! It is not as easy as it looks.'

Not everything was easy for Stephen either. On Friday 12 April 1991, he gave a demonstration of psychic surgery for students of healing at Stansted Hall, Essex. Gordon Higginson, the late, much loved and well respected President of the Spiritualist National Union (SNU) had invited him for the day. Unfortunately, the demonstration may have been a little too graphic and Gordon subsequently went in print questioning whether this was the 'spiritual' way forward, criticism which upset Stephen very deeply.

Then *Daily Star* reporter Steve Purcell visited Stephen with photographer Tony Sapiano and their article appeared on Friday 5 July 1991. It outlined how a new television series about the paranormal, Granada's *James Randi: Psychic Investigator*, which was to start later that month, 'heavily criticized' Stephen and his work. The programme featured James Randi, a magician who investigates psychic phenomena. He expressed amazement that Stephen was allowed to operate on people and a spokesman for the British Medical Association said, 'This sounds like a very dangerous practice.' An expert on blood added, 'You cannot say you have removed a clot just by showing clotted blood in a glass. This sounds like bunkum to me.'

Three days later, a centre-page spread appeared in the *Daily Star* in which Mr Randi gave a full account of his doubts about every aspect of the paranormal and suggested that many 'cured' patients never had any medical evidence that there was ever anything wrong with them in the first place.

In the end, of course, everyone has to make up their own mind and people like Mr Randi do contribute to the debate by putting the opposite argument, keeping genuine healers on their toes and exposing fraud which can bring more pain and misery to those who are already suffering. For this, he is to be commended, even if it may be hard to agree with some of his conclusions.

Mr Randi had not actually visited Stephen before he attacked his healing efforts on national television, although a research team, doctor and film crew had come to the clinic. Stephen and Kathy were then asked to travel to the TV studios in Manchester to 'defend themselves'. Significantly, the doctor who had accompanied the film crew to the clinic and been impressed by the work was left out of the programme in favour of another who had never been there, had not met Stephen before the day of the recording and had never seen the psychic surgeon in action. In spite of these rather hostile conditions, and perhaps due to some form of universal poetic justice, Stephen acquitted himself admirably and an incredible number of new enquiries resulted from this unsolicited national exposure.

Patients were even arriving by the coachload from Turkey. A Turkish journalist, Nevsal Elevi, had telephoned out of the blue and made an appointment to interview Stephen. She had been scheduled to have her womb removed in a Turkish hospital, but Dr Kahn offered to help and she later discovered that the problem had disappeared. Needless to say, given this experience, her subsequent article, published on 19 July 1991 in the Turkish newspaper *Hurryiett*, started a veritable avalanche of visitors from that part of the world.

One very sad aspect of this influx from the Near East was the large number of Kurdish people who had knife, bullet and shrapnel wounds from the conflict in that region. Very many had been tortured and the Turoffs and their spirit friends did all they could for these people, whose problems ranged from psychological trauma to very physical injuries, such as burnt testicles caused by the application of live electrodes during interrogation.

The end of July 1991 brought a series of problems for Stephen and Kathy. Like many healers, they have a very close affinity to animals and were sorry when on 25 July their cat Sam died. Then, the very next morning, Stephen pulled his back the wrong way getting out of a chair. With patients waiting, he worked in pain through the day and then left, with Kathy, for Bath, where they were due to give a weekend demonstration. After the long drive, he could hardly stand. He worked through the Saturday but by the evening the pain was so excruciating that he had to be taken to hospital.

'You've probably pulled a muscle,' said a young doctor as she went off to get the results of the X-ray.

'Don't move, Mr Turoff!' shouted a different, very senior-looking doctor as he marched briskly into the room, clutching the X-rays. 'Your back is broken! If you move an inch you may sever the spinal cord and be paralysed for the rest of your days.'

Not surprisingly, Stephen did not move a millimetre until a contraption and dressings were fitted to keep his back firmly in place All he could think about was his forthcoming healing diary.

'When will I be able to leave hospital and get back to my work?'

'I can't let you move, let alone out of the hospital,' replied the orthopaedic surgeon firmly.

'How long will I be in here?'

'Oh, six to 10 weeks in traction and then we will decide if we can risk operating.'

'Great. Just great.'

With a great deal on her mind, Kathy travelled back to Danbury the next day to be confronted with even more bad news: her grandmother had died just a few hours previously.

In hospital the following Wednesday, in pain and feeling low, Stephen turned on the TV to watch James Randi. It was the very programme which was critical of him. This made him feel even worse and he wondered what was the purpose of all these problems. Stephen is very much like the rest of us in that he often despairs at what life throws at him. Even though he is 100 per cent convinced that God's greater and higher purpose is being served at all times and in all places, he still wonders how during those periods when nothing seems to go right or make any sense.

To add to Stephen's problems, *Psychic News* then published details of loosely veiled criticisms that were now being made of his work by people in his own field. The heading read 'Surgeon defends using instruments' and the article began:

Healer Stephen Turoff last week defended the use of instruments during his psychic surgery. At the Spiritualist National Union's annual meeting (August 10), president Gordon Higginson spoke against the use of instruments when treating patients. Stephen was not named at the time. A week later, William Lang, the guide of trance healer George Chapman, also voiced concern, commenting, 'I feel that those people who are practising healing should do so the spiritual way.'

Stephen said: 'Though my name was not mentioned, it is quite obvious to whom they were referring. At present, I am the only psychic surgeon working with instruments in this country. While I am aware of the two outstanding mediums, Mr Chapman and Mr Higginson, and their contribution to the Spiritualist movement, it does not give them the right to attack another medium whose work has been tested throughout the world.'

When would all these problems end?

As if in answer, just five days after entering hospital, Stephen was out and about. The doctors could offer no medical explanation for this miraculous recovery.

Still, 1992 started as 1991 had finished – with more criticism. A front-page article in the 18 January issue of the Peterborough *Evening Post*, entitled 'Dead doc's £3 healing', read:

> *Church leaders today launched a scathing attack on a psychic group charging city people £3 to be healed by a spiritual doctor – who died 80 years ago. The display of spiritual healing is to be held in the city in March by a medium from Essex and involves 'psychic' operations carried out without anaesthetic ...*
>
> *The Church leaders in Peterborough warned the methods were highly dangerous. Bretton Baptist Church minister Chris Doig said: 'The only person who can really set people free is Jesus Christ. We're not saying these kinds of powers aren't real but they are very dangerous and can cause physical and psychological problems.'*

As with all things in life, there are differences of opinion. But one cleric who actually experienced the psychic surgery performed by Dr Kahn was Dennis Saint-Pierre, a Bishop of the Old Roman Catholic Church, who was affectionately known to Stephen as 'Father Dennis'. The Bishop's brother had contacted the healer in desperation when the cleric was in a hospice with stomach cancer and had been given just two weeks to live. Then Bishop Saint-Pierre himself asked Dr Kahn for help. 'I need 18 months in order to finish my mission here and settle my affairs,' he said. 'Can you give me that long?'

'As you know, my dear Bishop, it is God, and only God, who can give you more time. I will do what I can and, God willing, your wish will be granted.'

Bishop Saint-Pierre subsequently survived another 24 months with much reduced pain. Stephen got to know him over that period and some truly amazing developments transpired. Exorcisms, the Transfiguration of Christ onto Stephen's face and the independently verified appearance of stigmata on the cleric's hands and feet were some of the more major events which took place. But there were also a large number of less significant occurrences which ensured that his experiences with the Bishop would leave Stephen with enduring memories.

Bishop Saint-Pierre ordained Stephen as a healing minister of the Old Roman Catholic Church. He wanted to help with his healing mission and did whatever he could to contribute. One day, he was assisting in the clinic when a very troubled young man in his early twenties was brought in for healing. This poor unfortunate was possessed by a very dark entity which Stephen immediately recognized as requiring their joint and special attention – for an exorcism.

This is a very serious business and, with Stephen at the young man's head and Father Dennis at his feet, the entity began its attack. The big wooden crucifix dangling on a chain around the Bishop's neck began to spin slowly, backward and forward, forward and back. The victim initially began to shake until, suddenly, he started vibrating uncontrollably and, as the spinning of the cross became faster, so did the shaking of his body. An icy wind whirled around the room and Stephen and the Bishop stared at each other for support. Stephen closed his eyes and concentrated all his effort on the Light. The Bishop prayed. For 10 minutes the whirling wind, the body-shaking and the spinning of the cross continued. Then it all simply stopped, dying away as quickly as it had begun. The patient was calm, relaxed ... and healed.

'Look at me,' shouted Father Dennis, opening the palms of his hands for Stephen and the patient to see. 'I'm a marked man.' Quarter-inch wounds had appeared on his hands and, he found out later, also on his feet. Many others saw these marks and they remained with the Bishop until he passed on.

From the day he met Bishop Saint-Pierre, things began to look up for Stephen. He had renewed purpose and more energy to carry on in the face of continuing adversity:

> *It's almost as if Father Dennis was sent to me, at a very low point in my life, after a succession of knocks had got me down, and he put me back on the right road.*

Stephen and Kathy picked themselves up and got on with the healing work. On Saturday 18 August 1992 they demonstrated psychic surgery for Sutton Spiritualist church in the Birmingham area. Local journalist Pam Thompson wrote an article, 'Mum claims: "Tumour was cured by spirit surgery" ', which told how a young mother with a brain tumour was believed by doctors to have beaten the cancer after having been treated by Stephen. Her name was Val Brown and she wanted other sick people to experience the spirit surgery for themselves.

'People do not believe me when I tell them and I almost do not believe it myself. My logical mind cannot comprehend it and yet I was there and saw what he did,' she said.

Val's claim was backed by fellow Sutton Spiritualist church member Sue Brotherton, who said that Mr Turoff had cured her of a serious internal complaint. 'I have seen so many people helped over the years there is no doubt in my mind that Stephen is genuine,' she said.

Dr Sylvia Gyde, Director of Public Health for North Birmingham Health Authority, said, 'I think faith can do great things psychologically,' But she warned, 'If this man is going to cut into patients and actually draw blood, people should be very careful. Instruments should be clean and sterilized as we have problems of Hepatitis B and the Aids virus being spread through dirty instruments.'

According to Dr Kahn the spirit surgery team are sterilizing instruments on an etheric level and therefore no risk of infection has ever existed for the patients who are being cut open, but Dr Gyde's comments did point the way to a later decision by the spirit team to dematerialize the blood and other body tissues so that potential criticism of the psychic surgery in the modern Aids-conscious environment could be minimized.

Whatever the comments from the medical profession, patient satisfaction with Danbury Healing Clinic was enormous and there was more favourable media attention. An article by journalist Victoria Freeman in 31 August 1992 issue of *Woman* magazine created a great deal of interest. Publicity and personal recommendation from satisfied patients have ensured a steady growth in the numbers of people coming to Stephen. He has never advertised.

In 1992, a story broke which Stephen had been rather shy about mentioning. Three years earlier, he had received a knighthood from the Polish Government in exile for 'services rendered to humanity by spiritual healing, bringing hope and comfort to those who need it most'. Stephen had been introduced to Count Julius Sokoliniki, the President of the Republic of Poland, representing the Polish government in exile. His wife was very ill with a brain tumour and Stephen had helped her immensely. In honour of his healing and charitable work, he had been given a knighthood and his wife was made a Dame. Stephen's first idea was to turn it down, but various friends encouraged him to accept it and Dr Kahn agreed, so the honour was bestowed.

No strangers by now to working abroad, the Turoffs' next trip was back to the Dr Kahn Healing Centre in Fuengirola, Spain. A registered charity had now been set up and the centre was being run by director Esteban Molina and a growing team of willing helpers. The centre had grown enormously popular and at times police had been called to quell near riots outside.

'When the phone lines were open for my previous visit, 1,000 bookings were taken in three hours and many more had to be turned away,' explained Stephen. 'Unfortunately, this did not stop people turning up without appointments.' Bookings for the centre were being sold on the black market for £500 or more, while many people offered presents to the girls on reception. 'We didn't want this kind of thing,' Stephen added. 'Everything we do is free of charge. It is simply a matter of donations.'

There are days at the centre 'when the crippled and bedridden walk,' said Stephen. 'Dr Kahn, being the jolly fellow he is, often walks the patient outside to the waiting crowd and throws their sticks and crutches away.'

As the centre at Fuengirola was becoming too small, plans were being laid for another in the area of Coin, Malaga, as well as for the proposed orphanage. As Stephen told *Psychic News*:

> It's a huge project, it is due to take up four and a half acres of land and contain five healing rooms, ten bedrooms, a conference area, dining room, kitchen and, it is hoped, a chapel.
>
> There are also hopes to build an orphanage in the same area. Dedicated purely to spiritual healing, the new centre will be located on land we bought at a good price through a friend. Only later, after hearing stories from old people in the area and checking up in the town hall, did we discover the

*land around the new centre was known as 'The Hill
of the Miracle'.*

*It seems we'd been led out here by the spirit
world. Water has seeped out of the land where it
should not have been possible. A well on the side of
the hill filled immediately. There have been reports
of people rubbing this water into their skin and
being cured of many illnesses.*

Bishop Saint-Pierre blessed the land, an event which was
filmed by a group who are part of Paramount Pictures. Then,
when a large white cross was erected at the site, there were
reports of a lamb materializing next to it.

'There was a thicket by the white cross which the lamb
ran into,' said Stephen. 'This was searched, but the lamb had
just disappeared. There was nowhere else for it to go.'

A further phenomenon was the sighting of strange lights
which appeared over the cross. According to Stephen, 'This
information came from the wife of one of the film crew who
visited the hill. She was not a Spiritualist. The site was rather
inaccessible but a bridge has now been placed over the river in
the valley below. Electrical pylons have also been built on the
land. It was as though people had been manipulated into getting something done.' Many in the nearby village pledged
their support for the planned centre.

I visited Fuengirola in August 1995 to interview Esteban
and to see the progress of the new Dr Joseph Kahn Healing
Centre. At time of writing (July 1996) it is half-finished. It has
five healing rooms, a large waiting area and space allocated for
a 60-bed orphanage. It is a 3-acre site set against the hillside.
All around the front is a tree-lined walkway which will be
dedicated to the world's main religions. A shrine dedicated to
'The Nazarene' will feature at the end of the walkway. The
site affords panoramic views of the surrounding mountains

and the Mediterranean coastline. I search for an adequate word to describe it all: *biblical*.

The water will be supplied by a well which was found by Antonio, a diviner who says he is 'guided by the Virgin'. He is used by the local government when they want to look for water at various sites. He picked a spot. They drilled down 30 metres (100 ft) and found water. He said drill deeper. At 70 metres (230 ft) they tapped a second stream. The diviner said drill deeper still. At 90 metres (300 ft), a third stream was found. Half-a-litre per second of water supply is considered good in this arid region of southern Spain. Thanks to the diviner, the Dr Joseph Kahn Healing Centre will benefit from 5 litres per second! Dr Kahn has told Esteban Molina that the centre will be huge, 'bigger than Lourdes' one day.

However, as Stephen said in 1992:

Spain is a problem country for healers. I feel many people don't realize the dangers of practising here. It is advisable to be a charity. You are not supposed to work without a work permit. You can get locked up for healing in Spain. If someone comes and is not happy they can go to the police and denounce you. Then you have to prove your innocence.

This turned out to be a prophetic insight.

In February 1993, an official complaint was received from the Medical Association in Malaga. They had interpreted various newspaper and magazine articles as evidence that Stephen was purporting to be a doctor. A picture in the local press, of scissors being fully inserted into a patient's nose, was the final straw. Stephen was in the country at the time and was summoned to appear before a local judge to answer the allegations.

'Have you been taking drugs, Mr Turoff?' she asked him. 'Have you banged your head recently?'

Things did not look good when she decided that Stephen would have to submit to tests with the police psychiatrist. He was to be detained in custody until the psychiatrist could certify him fit to practise. Meantime, over 900 people were in the appointment book for the coming week. They were due to arrive from all over Spain. Many had booked accommodation to stay overnight.

Finally, after many hours in court and being interviewed by the police psychiatrist, Stephen was told by the judge that he was free to go and that no action would be taken at that time. Stephen and Kathy left the court and hired a good lawyer, who advised them not to practise until the court had agreed they could continue to do so. They returned home, leaving all the patients untreated.

Interestingly, Dr Kahn told Esteban to start healing and prepare himself to do the psychic surgery at the same time as Stephen was being stopped from doing so. Esteban's gift developed rapidly, almost overnight.

The following article, from the Christmas 1993 issue of *Psychic News*, gives some idea of the problems of working in Spain:

15 MILLION SEE PSYCHIC SURGEON RESTORE SIGHT

Patient Produces Medical Records to Disprove Accusations of Fraud

A woman who regained the sight of her left eye after psychic surgery has been forced to produce medical records on television to crush accusations of fraud.

Isabel Duran from Madrid had a spirit operation on the Spanish television discussion programme Otra Dimension.

Presented by Felix Gracia, the show featured interviews with both Danbury, Essex, healer Stephen Turoff and Dr Joseph Kahn, the spirit physician who works through Stephen's entranced body.

It also hosted an extensive demonstration of psychic surgery. Dr Kahn was seen using various instruments on patients. It made gruesome viewing at times, but sufferers were clearly not in any pain during the operations.

Isabel was among the first to be treated. She was blind in her left eye. But after healing, she could see with it and was later filmed – her right eye covered up – reading a newspaper.

Unfortunately, it seems that not all of the estimated 15 million viewers who watched the programme found the demonstration inspiring.

Speaking from his Danbury clinic, Stephen told PN that the show sparked off new attempts by the Spanish medical profession to ban his work.

'On top of this,' he added, 'the newspapers were full of claims that I had actually paid the woman to say she was blind before embarking on the spirit operation.'

Indeed, only when Isabel returned to the programme and held up medical records proving her condition did the accusations of fraud stop...

As he described the events which led up to his appearance, Mr Turoff admitted that he needed strong persuasion in light of the unfair way he has been treated in the past.

'For some time a Spanish magazine on the paranormal has been printing articles about me,' explained the healer.

'They arranged a test for Dr Kahn's healing, but

brought along nothing but mentally-retarded chil-
dren as patients, so it was hardly fair.

'Nevertheless, the results were good and I was
later asked to become entranced on Otra Dimension.*'*

Due to popular demand, this edition of *Otra Dimension* has
been repeated six times on Spanish national television.

In Britain, medical records have until recently not been
available to patients, making it difficult to show the difference before and after healing. Now people are able to have
access to their records, perhaps we will one day see a serious
study of the effects of psychic surgery. In the interests of fur-
thering knowledge, Stephen is ready and willing to take part
in this sort of study. All he needs is an equally willing group
of patients and doctors.

Back in Spain, in November 1993, Stephen's lawyer and
Esteban Molina arrived at the court with Stephen's book,
videos of psychic surgery in progress and other evidence in
support of Stephen's right to practise. The judge saw no reason
why Stephen should not offer healing and psychic surgery to
the public and the case was dismissed. Stephen returned in
February 1994 to take up where he had left off.

In 1995, when I asked Esteban to put an estimate on the
number of patients who had been through the centre since it
all started, he replied, 'Well over 20,000.'

Meantime, the Danbury Healing Clinic seemed to be having
an influence on other healers. As well as receiving healing,
they seemed to go away with a greater enthusiasm for giving
healing to others. One healer, the author of *This Gift Is Not
for Me*, wrote:

Dear Stephen and Kathy,

Many thanks for a wonderful afternoon spent with you and Dr Kahn ... Having embarked on psychic surgery myself, Stephen, Dr Kahn's demonstration showed me a side ... I haven't witnessed before! All power to you and all our wonderful spirit helpers and guides!

... Who knows, Stephen, perhaps one day we shall work together (having been told many years ago that I would be working in Spain)?

I enjoyed your book very much. Glad to know you enjoyed mine, Kathy. I doubt if Stephen gets much time to read.

All kind thoughts & God bless

Margaret Collier

However, the people living in the West Belvedere cul-de-sac in Danbury village were becoming a bit tired of hordes of people descending on the area and parking on the verges and corners. Even though many local people were sympathetic towards the desperate plight of some of the patients who were coming to Stephen for help, and many were patients themselves, it is perhaps understandable that the daily invasion would put out the neighbours.

At one time the local authorities sent a team of councillors to inspect what was happening. I had taken some friends to the clinic that day and had been asked to ensure that visitors parked in the right place. On seeing a car pull up and park right outside on the verge, I went down the path and politely asked the driver: 'Would you mind parking along the road as the council are doing an inspection today?'

'We *are* the council team,' said the driver and, rather strangely, elected to leave his car right where the neighbours were likely to complain about it! Needless to say, my contribution had not furthered the cause and I was never asked to be car park attendant again.

The council suggested that using another venue might be a good idea and some time later, the sheer volume of patients coming from all over the world necessitated the leasing of a suite of rooms at the Miami Hotel in Chelmsford. Visitors now have the benefit of the hotel car park and restaurant and accommodation facilities if required. Sometimes whole groups come to stay at the hotel. They can simply walk across the courtyard when it is time for their appointment.

Despite all the apparent successes, no healer claims to be able to help everyone and sometimes those closest to the healer are the ones they are least able to help. Kitty, Stephen's mother, was in considerable pain with ulcers on her legs for 12 years, but whilst Stephen did all he could to help, the condition continued to trouble her until her death, early in 1994, of a heart attack. At the funeral service, held in the Enfield Crematorium, Stephen's sisters told me that they and Stephen shared the front pew. All had gone as expected until a shaft of bright white light streamed through the high windows and bathed the three of them, just as the coffin was disappearing through the doors. This event, on an otherwise dull and dreary day, was sufficiently remarkable to draw comment.

It was a short while later that the 'finger of God' photographic phenomena began. Stephen had prayed for God to show his light at the healing clinic and from the next day onwards, beautiful pastel lights began appearing on photographs taken there. Ordinary people took ordinary photographs with ordinary cameras, but the lights in the pictures were quite extraordinary.

Later, they began appearing on photographs wherever Stephen travelled around the world.

These extraordinary lights marked the beginning of another phase in Stephen Turoff's life and work. He believes that the lights, and all the other phenomena surrounding him, are caused by, and are directly attributable to, his ever-present spiritual guide and mentor, Sathya Sai Baba.

Stephen first came to know of Sai Baba in his mid twenties. This 'national treasure of India' is, on first impression, a little man with a large crown of black crinkly hair. He seldom sleeps. He has an incredible sense of humour. At the age of 13, he declared that he was an avatar, an incarnation of God on Earth. His clearly stated tasks are simple: to avoid the destruction, by humankind, of our physical home, Mother Earth, and to show us the way back to our true Home, to God. He now has many millions of devotees in India, together with thousands of Sai Centres, as well as colleges, universities and hospitals, and there are Sai Centres in virtually every country of the Western world.

Sai Baba has performed many miracles, which he calls mere 'calling cards', toys and tricks to gain our interest and to demonstrate the illusion of our physical bodies and the material world to which we are all so attached. These miracles include producing sacred ash, which he calls *vibhuti*, from thin air or empty urns. He sprinkles it over his followers and visitors and tells people to eat it to cure sickness. Today, millions of people have had experiences of *vibhuti* forming in their places of worship or even in their homes. It is now constantly manifesting at Stephen's clinic, where he rubs it into the patients' affected area or gives it to people to eat.

The number and range of Sathya Sai Baba's miracles has increased over the years. These phenomena are, however, nothing when compared to his ability to teach and spread a spiritual message, the underlying principle of which is Divine Love.

This message has deeply influenced Stephen's own life.

5

CHANGE:
THE SPIRITUAL TEACHER

If one student is bad, only that student is affected.
But if one teacher is bad, hundreds of students get
spoiled.

SAI BABA

The good teacher teaches steadily and carefully:
thoughts affect karma; words affect karma; actions
affect karma.

DR KAHN

Teaching comes through me, not from me.

STEPHEN TUROFF

'I died in the Battle of the Somme,' said James Legget, a First
World War soldier, as he came through loud and clear to
Stephen's audience at the end of 1985. It was a cold November
morning, Remembrance Sunday, and Stephen was demon-
strating clairvoyance at Sudbury church in Suffolk. Over the
next two years, James communicated with Stephen on a regular basis and the result was *Seven Steps to Eternity* (Elmore-
Chard, 1987), a book which tells the story of the soldier's
death and his life thereafter in spirit. Stephen says he finds
writing difficult – 'I can't string two words together, let alone
two sentences' – and yet he considers putting the book together one of his most rewarding experiences.

Reviewer Danny Ansell, in 4 November issue of *Psychic News*, agreed:

> *Although literally crammed with spiritual truths and teachings, the story remains consistent and illuminating throughout ... a refreshing sense of humour is maintained ... One of the best books of this genre to cross my desk in some time, its easy style will be of equal appeal to experienced readers and newcomers to spiritual matters alike.*

Seven Steps to Eternity probably marked the beginning of Stephen's development as a spiritual teacher. As he explains in the preface:

> *As a psychic, I have been privileged to have numerous encounters with astral-dwelling souls. They have enlightened me in every sense of the word about their experiences in the planes after death.*
>
> *When a soul first leaves his body, he falls into a sleep-like state and awakens on the plane of the astral world suitable for him. I am often questioned about this term 'plane' and the nearest answer is a 'state' of vibration. For example, sound waves; ultraviolet waves from the sun; rays from an electric lamp; all of these are invisible, each interpenetrating, yet do not affect or interfere with each other. So it is with the planes in the astral world.*
>
> *Dwelling on each plane are the souls appropriate to live and operate there according to their spiritual evolution: 'In My Father's House there are many mansions.'*
>
> *...One day [James] asked if I would consider writing a book about his life, not his tragically short*

*one on our plane, but in the planes he has moved
through since passing.*

After Jim's 'death', he is met by 'officers' who help him get
used to his new surroundings. Officers, of course, would be
familiar to a soldier and this would reduce the initial shock
and aid the transition to the next world. Some time later, Jim
is ready to begin learning about his new life and is taken to a
'church-like' building:

> *We went inside and took our seats. In front of us was
> an altar, table and two chairs ... Suddenly a whirling
> mist appeared from nowhere. It began to shape itself
> into the form of a man and shimmered from head to
> foot as it solidified. In front of us stood a man where
> only a moment ago was empty space ...*
>
> *'Obviously, I have your attention,' said the
> teacher. 'I can't think of a better way of getting that
> than an impressive entrance. First, I want to speak
> to you about your new environment. You are on the
> fourth of seven astral planes. Each plane differs from
> the others by the manifestation, density, and veloci-
> ty of its basic essence. Your physical body varies in a
> way that determines your spiritual growth, which is
> what your soul is always seeking. Many of you liter-
> ally starve your souls and, for example, allow your
> minds to become entirely engrossed and dominated
> by materialism.*
>
> *'The soul is always called on to look up, not
> back. It must carry hope and love at the helm of
> your life. This is not always easy ... yet to make an
> effort is always a step in the right direction.*
>
> *... You have been told there are seven planes.
> Likewise you have seven bodies. One of these was*

the physical body which you discarded when you left the earth plane. Here on the fourth astral plane, your astral body is learning to vibrate in accordance with the vibrations here. These are finer and faster than those on the earth plane. This explains why things here are as tangible and real as on earth ... As the third and fourth planes are only slightly finer than the earth plane, it is our endeavour that you move to the fifth plane. This will occur when you refine your mental and emotional vibrations. I come from the seventh plane where matter vibrates faster and is more refined than here.

'You may wonder how I am able to visit your plane ... I have learned to wind down my vibrations in order to work on the lower planes ... by the power of thought.'

Then the captain took questions from the audience.

'Is there a God, sir?'

'Yes there is a God and we will explain later about the God force which is within all things.'

'Will I be able to see my wife and talk to her, sir?'

'You ... will be allocated a special guide who will teach you how to communicate with your loved ones.'

Shortly afterwards, Jim meets his guide, an 800-year-old Chinese gentleman who, like Stephen's guide, is named Chan:

I looked him up and down and admired his splendid clothes. The colours were vivid as though they were alive. I wondered where he was from. 'From the sixth plane, where I live, of course,' he said.

'Hey, I never spoke. How did you know what I was thinking?'

'I can read your thoughts,' he answered. 'Here it's not necessary to speak. You too will learn to use your higher senses for speech ... You are taken through the astral planes in stages. Each one educates you for the next. You will have to readjust your old idea of earth schooling, but I will be your teacher ...

'Your first lesson will be to learn how to focus your thoughts by concentrating your willpower. You can then communicate with other souls mentally. The way this works is that a Thought becomes the Line, and the Will becomes the Impulse.

... Now then, Jim. I want to talk to you about your sleeping habits ... You will find many beneficial changes here. One is that you will require no sleep ... Many think that all their troubles will disappear with a night's sleep. Nothing is further from the truth. Do you realize you have spent a third of your life asleep? At times you will find it necessary to rest in order to digest what you have learnt, but sleep as you have known it will be unnecessary.'

... He asked if I had any other questions.

'Yes,' I replied. 'Where can I get something to eat? I'm bloody starving.'

'I was waiting for that,' he teased. 'Do you remember what I was saying a moment ago, about sleep? Well, the same thing applies to eating ... There is a good reason for this. The conditions of life on the higher spheres are more dependent on mental power than those of the earth plane ... You have a body which is a duplicate of the one you had on the earth plane ... but [it is] not used in the same way as on

the earth plane because here you do not eat coarse
food which must be processed ... Here we absorb
food or fuel through the pores of our skin as well as
through our breath. This is totally adequate for our
well-being.'

Initially, all the teachings from Dr Kahn, Jim and Chan were
'channelled' ideas and thoughts. At this time, Dr Kahn was
taking over Stephen's body completely for up to eight hours a
day. In that deep trance state, it was Dr Kahn and not Stephen
who would talk to people, give them words of wisdom, occasionally pass on messages from 'dead' relatives and so on.
After coming out of trance, Stephen would go home, have his
meal and sit back in his chair to meditate. This allowed Jim
and Chan to 'place pictures' in his head, every night, for two
years whilst he wrote the book. So Stephen was being used as
an 'instrument' for the teaching that was coming through in
much the same way as he was an instrument for the healing.

Dr Kahn continued with the deep trance control until
1991, when the younger Dr Kahn was able to come through.
The second Dr Kahn was able to use Stephen's body in a 'light
trance'. This enabled Stephen to be in full command of his
own faculties and meant that he could give people advice
himself, with the benefit of the spirit team's ability to communicate with a patient's higher self. As already mentioned,
it was essential for Stephen's own development to take a conscious part in the healing and teaching process.

In November 1992, *Options* magazine interviewed Stephen
and five other well known psychics. In this interview Stephen
explains something of his development:

Beginnings

'I used to hear voices and see colours around people ... I'd hear voices telling me things. I saw doctors and opticians to get help. People thought I was schizophrenic. But I found a Spiritualist church and they explained that I was in tune with another dimension.'

Developing the Skills

'The healing power started as soon as I accepted the voices existed and what they were saying was real. They told me I was a healer and I began to cure people. I had no formal health training ...'

How It Works

'I'm different to other healers, in that I actually perform surgery ... An external personality takes me over ... I don't even know what I'm doing.'

Spiritual Guides

'We have one overall guide – a guardian angel if you like – and the others will appear from time to time to enhance your particular gifts. Doctor Kahn has enhanced the healing gift and I have a Chinese gentleman giving me philosophy ...'

A Logical Explanation?

'The established medical world would prefer to forget me. They sent a doctor here who watched me dematerialize a woman's eye, do some work in the socket, and rematerialize it again. I can't even explain that myself, so how do you expect a doctor to? I don't know – ignorance is bliss for me.'

A Blessing or a Curse?
'It's been a blessing, but I don't know why I was chosen. In most ways, I'm just an ordinary person.'

In order to enlighten people further as to the healing team's work and mission, Dr Kahn conducted a question and answer session with a journalist from *Psychic News* in September 1992. He told how he physically 'shrinks' his medium in order to treat patients and Stephen corroborated this, commenting that, in comparison to his own large stature, 'Dr Kahn is a very small man. When I come out of trance, it can be very painful.' Dr Kahn explained that the work depleted Stephen's physical body, so he needed to take vitamins and mineral supplements daily. Other spirit surgeons were also seeking 'instruments' with whom to work on the physical plane, but they needed to be people with both great strength of character and the ability to become psychic surgeons. Sensitivity was important.

When asked what life was like in the spirit world, he said:

I come from the seventh sub-plane of the astral world, just before the Wall of Fire where matter ceases to exist. I am using the body of Dr Kahn. I keep Dr Kahn alive by leaving a portion of my consciousness within his frame. If I were to withdraw all consciousness from that astral body, then it would go back to the natural elements and I would not be able to communicate with you. The rest of me is spirit. I would not want to go back to Earth permanently. I would not be able to cope with it now. When you come to my side of life you will realize why. You have many words saying how beautiful our spheres are, but you will not know it until you come here.

He added, 'There is much change to take place in your world and it is going to be drastic change. It has already begun.'

Dr Kahn also shared some of his knowledge and thoughts with Mark, Kathy's son, who was very interested in the work being done:

> Dr Kahn, can you cast any light on the subject of reincarnation, and at what stage does the soul enter the body?
>
> *'I will answer the second part of your question first.*
>
> *'When the ovum or female germ-cell is fertilized by the male sperm, there is an instantaneous formation of protoplasm of microscopic size. It is this formation, as you would understand it, that is termed physical life. The soul does not enter after this formation, because the soul essence has already established itself in the first formation. The most striking characteristic of protoplasm is its ability to change shape and position, by some intrinsic power. The cause of this is by way of a nuclear matrix. The matrix is a minute body, embedded in the protoplasm, giving the protoplasm its orders for shape, size and intelligence. From the very instant the ovum has been fertilized by male sperm, an etheric counterpart of the cell structure takes place. Thus the cells form themselves into a foetus with the etheric foetus being formed in just the same manner.*
>
> *... As for reincarnation, there is but one diamond with many facets... We are all parts of one whole, all working in unison. There is no "personal" self. Your "persona" or player's mask will be dropped*

with your present garb of flesh when you leave your Earth. But your entity – your individual, independent, distinctive character – will remain, not as a separated "thing", but as a quality related to the whole.'

... How is it that some people can remember what they term 'past lives'?

We are all consciously, or unconsciously, striving to find our way back to the Divine from which we sprang. Matter has its own stage of development and is therefore "spiritualized" by past incoming souls who have left a knowledge of how to manage the transition.

'As your spirit takes more control of its new body, it also takes control of the recording process of past experiences in its previous expressions ... so in fact, when a person says they have lived before in a previous life as a Chinaman, or princess, this is somewhat incorrect.

'What they have discovered is the true art of psychometry, the art of holding an object and "reading" it ...'

How does this correspond with physical difficulties? I have heard it said that disabilities relate to 'karma'.

The matrix automatically draws protoplasm unto itself that will correspond to the information passed on to it by the higher state of expression, the soul's group activity and need for learning ... [So] you must not look down upon those with a disability because they themselves have been party to its design.'

How then can you cure the sick if it is their destiny to suffer?

'We first have to see if the illness is part of the karmic pattern, or if it is an incoming disease. If the former, then we ... have to talk to the higher self of the patient to see what stage it has reached in its development. If the patient has not yet learned from his condition, then we are unable to intervene, but that does not mean that all is lost. For, in truth, it is the patient who, by deep prayer and meditation, may come to terms with his physical disability and allow God to enter his life ...

'Now to that which you call "disease". One of the greatest causes of dis-ease today is stress ... When "disharmony", in any sense of the word, disturbs the harmonic vibrations of the senses, the brain immediately starts to react ... and stress occurs.

'To understand how these vibrations work, we must look at the operation of ... the Law of Rhythmic Breath and its corresponding influence upon the physical body. The universal current of life, or vital force, which pervades all space and is commonly recognized in the body as breath, is compounded of atoms, or electrons, which are differentiated by their characteristic motions into five forms of vibrations.

'Your scientists have so far recognized only two of these subtle ethers and have not yet discovered their profound influence upon all living things. But on saying this, the scientists are now on the verge of a much greater discovery; and that is sub-atomic physics. This will eventually prove without doubt the existence of the next dimension.

'... Each of the five vibrations is a force of motion and each is both "substance" and "force". I will give you their common names for future reference: the sound vibration [we can hear]; the tangiferous vibration [we can touch]; the luminiferous ether [we can see]; the gustiferous ether [we can taste] and the odiferous ether [we can smell].

'Each of these five energies has its positive and negative phases throughout the cosmos. In normal health, their flow and proportion vary from time to time with absolute rhythmic precision. It is only when this rhythm is disrupted that we see its effect for good or ill. Every disease is any influence that disturbs nature's intricate but symmetrical balance of these etheric life forces...

'To gain a balanced body and mind, you must learn to control the breath and the vital forces that flow in and throughout the whole physical body and to allow only harmonious energies to be transmuted into positive life force.'

If the higher self has learnt from its disability, what then happens if that person does not come into contact with a healer?

'First let me say that there are no such things as coincidences in life.'

So where does free will come into it, Joseph?

'Let me answer your first question. If you have a disability, and are ready to be healed, no matter what the lower self decides, the higher self will set in motion the correct pathway that you should take. If you are uncertain how to act, do not fret about it. Do not let your mind be troubled and disturbed by doubts. Just take the difficulty or the question, lay it before the Higher Power and pray that you may be *shown the right direction. This is where your free will comes into operation – to use your willpower as a positive implement in your quest for health.'*

What attitude should we have when we near the end of our days?

'Happiness. Happiness is an uplifting force only equalled by the sun's rays. It is sunshine in the heart! And it moves with a joyous rhythm that sings through the body. Therefore, no medicine in the pharma-copoeia possesses the curative virtue of happiness.'

Our attitude towards physical death should then be one of expectancy and looking forward to the great day of our release?

'Your soul is already getting ready for its transi-tion. Nightly your soul leaves its physical body when you lie down to rest and joins with those of my world … The spirit goes into the higher regions and gathers vital forces and magnetism with which it returns and revives the body.'

What then happens at the deathbed?

'The separation of the etheric body from the inert physical body … The etheric double is the form around which the physical body is built and is made up of the etheric matter which will live and breathe in the etheric world. The separation is an easing out of the etheric atoms. These two bodies are connected by the Cord of Light. When death occurs, the physi-cal consciousness is transferred through the cord to the etheric brain. Then, and only on the complete separation of these two bodies, does the Cord of Light cease to exist.'

So why do some people who have had near-death experiences say that they have felt themselves going through a tunnel and seen a light at the end of it?

'Consciousness is transferred through the cord to the etheric brain. This transference is the tunnel of which you speak. The etheric eyes are the light at the end of the tunnel which connect to the etheric wavelength as it adjusts to its new world.'

Before we end, Joseph, can you give us some words of encouragement?

'We speak to you in words once again, but we have often spoken to you in the silence of your own sanctuary. When the battle of life and the noise of the world clang around you, we are helping you to guide your ship over the rough waters. When at times the canvas is hauled down and your ship is running with bare masts before the wind, she is not deserted; the storms and waves that buffet her are but the forces instrumental in bringing her nearer to port.'

Just like the rest of us, Stephen is growing, developing and changing spiritually. Here are some of his thoughts, which are extracts from a speech given on Sunday 13 August 1995 in Wolverhampton to 1,600 devotees of Sathya Sai Baba:

We should listen when our heart and our conscience tell us the truth. For who is it that speaks to us in that quiet inner voice, unless it is God?

God gives us 24 hours in a day. We should set aside 24 minutes of each day: eight minutes in the morning, eight minutes in the afternoon and eight minutes in the evening to listen to our quiet inner voice ... Try it and see what happens.

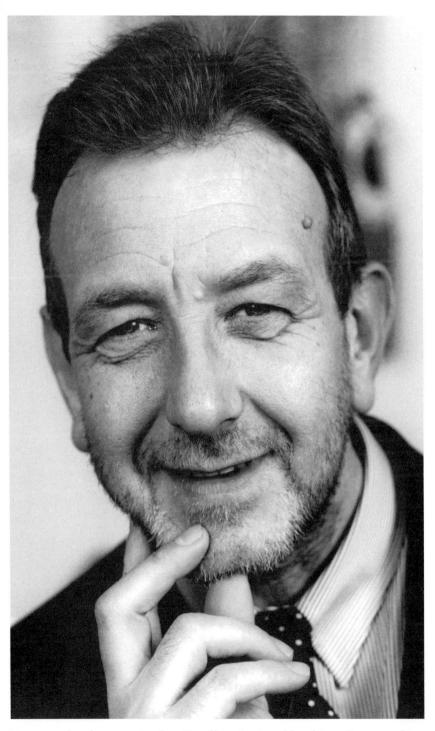

Many people who meet Stephen Turoff are intrigued by this ordinary working man who speaks with the wisdom of an Indian sage. © *Tim Caranagh*

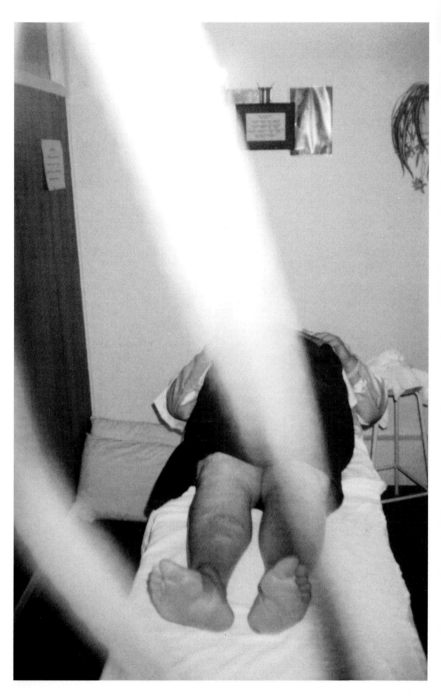

When Stephen works, beautiful pastel lights descend like lightning bolts from

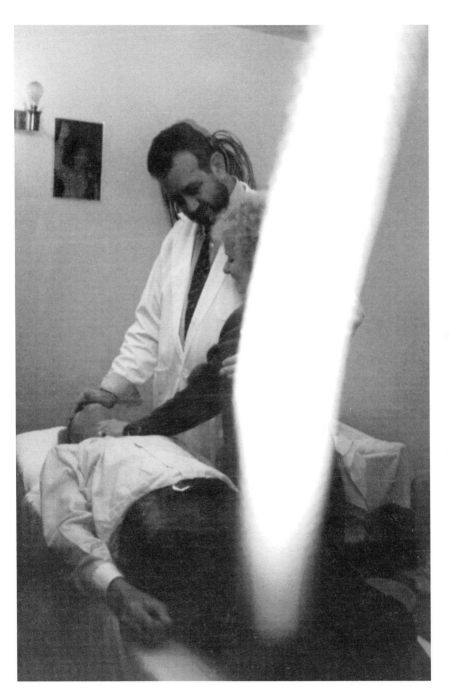

the sky into patients' bodies. He calls this phenomenon 'the finger of God'.

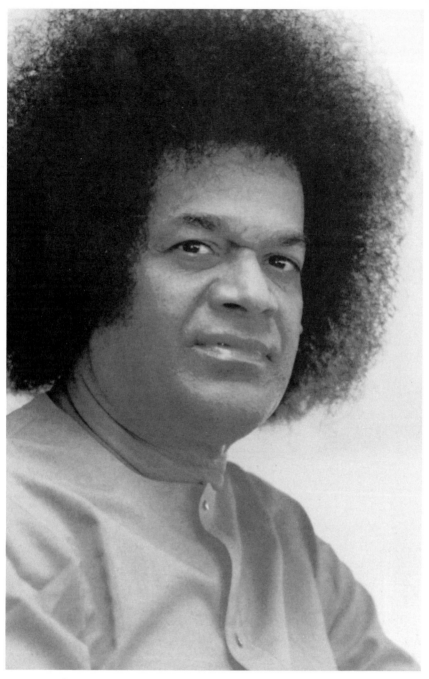

Sathya Sai Baba, the Indian mystic often called 'the man of miracles' has
influenced Stephen's work in fascinating ways. Sai Baba says, 'I am always
guarding you and guiding you. March on, have no fear.'

When you feel the distraction of the world or of people disturbing your poise, stop a moment, take a deep breath and quickly claim the strength of the divine within you. This will give you poise and renew your power to overcome the difficulty ... It is intended that you should gather strength by conquering difficulties ...

If you allow any condition to irritate you, you cease to be the master and this must not be. These seemingly irritating experiences and apparent stumbling blocks are for you to overcome; they are aids to your spiritual development.

If you feel at times that your environment hampers your own spiritual advance, that thought or feeling is a mistake. If you are tempted to think that you have failed in following your ideal ... abide in your place; you are strong enough to rise above even your most fanciful failures. The greatest lessons ... in the school of Earth-life come through the so-called failures.

... By the exercise of your free will, close the doors of your nature to all undeveloped forces. Do not admit ... fear or doubt, self-love, envy, hate, jealousy, indolence or ignorance. These are destructive forces which tear down and destroy. They put you out of tune so that you do not vibrate in harmony with God's plan.

... If you cannot deal with people who appear to be overwhelmed by the destructive forces, wish them well and give them back to God. For He is the all-seeing, all-knowing Master and it is He alone who can put them back on the right path.

Go out into the world among people, carrying the powerful love atmosphere which comforts and

heals the sick and suffering. Radiate peace and hap-
piness ... teach those who have not yet found the
love, truth and peace that is knowledge of God.
... God wants you, He needs you, as an instru-
ment in your own sphere, to bring others to an awak-
ening into soul-life.

Stephen's spiritual message appears to be based on a simple premise: actions speak louder than words. As Sai Baba says, 'Hands that help are holier than lips that pray.' Stephen acts on this himself, sending, for example, a percentage of his income directly to various causes. Indian farmers have received farm equipment and many other people have benefited from direct help. Stephen also presents himself and his work to anyone and everyone who is prepared to take some time to listen or take a look. All the phenomena surrounding him are occurring daily at the Danbury Healing Clinic and around the world wherever he visits. Everyone is welcome to go along to see, to experience and to decide for themselves.

Stephen simply believes he is doing God's work and he does it, day in and day out, to the best of his ability. He readily admits that his best is sometimes sadly lacking, but he is working on it. He often finishes a day wondering whether he can cope with tomorrow morning when another hundred or so very sick people will come to him expecting miracle solutions, but he carries on. Of his detractors he says, 'There will always be those who knock and mock. It is all part of the illusion, the experience, the mystery. None are right or wrong, they just are what they are. Each of us is having our own individual life experience and it is part of the knockers or mockers' experience to be and do exactly as they are and act.'

'Knockers and mockers' might also like to consider two laws that Stephen's spirit helpers often teach. The first is the

Law of Karma, which is summed up pretty well by the 'sow and reap' analogy. What you put out, you get back. What goes around, comes around.

The second law to consider is the Law of Perfection. The only person that we are able to perfect is ourselves. That is our task. Stephen asks, 'Why waste time, literally lifetimes, criticizing another soul's best efforts when you are not even attempting to perfect yourself first? Do not hinder others' efforts. Do not be too quick to judge. On the other hand, do all you can to help others and you will find you are helping yourself. If you understand the ultimate goal and simple rules of the game, playing is so much more fun, so much more rewarding and so much easier.'

'What is the simplest advice you could give for balancing karma and achieving perfection?' I ask in a quiet moment with Stephen. He sits back and thinks carefully ...

'See good, do good, be good.'

6

HEALING HAPPENS

'Miracle': a marvellous event occurring within
human experience which cannot have been
brought about by human power or by the operation of any natural agency, and must therefore be
ascribed to the special intervention of the Deity
or of some supernatural being: chiefly an act (e.g.
of healing) exhibiting control over the laws of
nature, and serving as evidence that the agent is
either divine or is specially favoured by God.

OXFORD ENGLISH DICTIONARY

The word 'healing' is derived from an ancient Anglo-Saxon
term meaning 'to make whole'. Many healers believe that this
wholeness is comprised of the four aspects of the human
being – the physical, the mental, the emotional and the spiritual. In this view, all of these aspects interact and not until
they are all in balance and harmony with each other and their
environment is 'healing' or 'wholeness' achieved.

Many other people believe that we are merely physical
beings, the highest order of the animals in a mechanical
world, and that our mental, emotional and even spiritual
capabilities are derived from our bio-chemical systems and
processes in a way that is yet to be fully understood.

Irrespective of their views, it is amazing the number of
people who will declare an interest in healing miracles in general, and psychic surgery in particular, given half a chance.

When I suggested to my brother-in-law, Rob Bennett, that he and his wife Veronica might like to have an evening of psychic surgery videos, I was fairly tentative and expected 'You must be joking' or, knowing Rob, something rather less polite.

'Why not?' he said. 'There's got to be more to life than we understand. It should be interesting.'

Picking myself up off the floor, I went home and a few hours later my wife Jane and I went back to their house with a Tesco's bag full of videos and got settled in with a beer and a take-away curry. Excepting the rather graphic eye-operations, which they just could not continue to watch, both Robbie and Ronnie were fascinated.

Next morning, we were having tea at Jane's parents' house and were told that Robbie had been describing the videos to one of the customers in his shop. To his surprise the customer said she had actually had psychic surgery performed by Brazilian Lourival de Freitas many years before. She had never needed any further treatment for the problem.

This made me wonder how many more closet psychic surgery enthusiasts there might be out there, people who would be interested in treatment if a reliable friend or relative said it was worth a try. After all, it *is* an attractive idea – no hospital waiting list, no anaesthetic, no drugs, little or no blood, relatively little pain, no side-effects, no disfiguring scars, no long recuperation and no time off work. Despite all these advantages, however, it might be some time before people routinely choose to complement their orthodox medical treatment with healing and/or psychic surgery. One reason for this might be the attitude of many in the medical establishment.

As mentioned previously, all the healing and other phenomena surrounding Stephen Turoff and his clinic are open to scrutiny by anyone who cares to take a look. It seems unfortunate that some medical people, including Nobel prize winners, choose *not* to investigate healing and other 'holistic' therapies but nevertheless speak out against them.

Nobel prizes, comprehensive research facilities and huge industry and governmental funding continue to be awarded to orthodox scientists, while less conventional ideas and methods of alleviating human sickness and suffering have not, in recent history at least, been afforded the same advantages. A great deal of research is, however, being done into complementary medicine in general and healing in particular. As already mentioned, in the early seventies, when Stephen was first developing his healing work, the efficacy of healing was being scientifically investigated by Professor Krieger in the United States. In 1993, the UK's respected *Nursing Times* outlined Professor Krieger's Therapeutic Touch:

> *Therapeutic Touch has a theoretical framework devised by Martha Rogers, also a nurse. It was ... based on well-documented research by biochemists, who examined the inexplicable results that 'healers' produced in wounded animals, and the growth of barley under strictly controlled conditions. (Dr Robert Miller was astounded to discover that when 'healers' concentrated on barley from 600 miles away, it grew 840% faster than the control barley.)*
>
> *Practitioners ... consider that human beings are energy fields, and an integral part of a 'universal life force' that extends beyond the physical body and interacts with everything in the environment. They believe that health is a manifestation of the free flow of this vital energy through the body, and that, conversely, ill-health results when there are problems with the energy flow. Therapeutic Touch practitioners claim to be able to attune themselves to this energy and to be able to help alter its flow to restore*

health. Although the word 'touch' is used ... skin-to-skin contact is not necessary for the fields to interact, as they extend beyond the skin's surface.

After Professor Krieger's first study, which, as already mentioned, appeared to demonstrate that Therapeutic Touch raised haemoglobin levels, she went on to publish another study in 1975. Her first study had been criticized to some extent in its design and controls by other scientists and the second study took account of their suggestions. It also showed the efficacy of Therapeutic Touch. In her book, *The Therapeutic Touch* (Prentice-Hall, 1979), Krieger gives case histories that feature conditions as varied as 'pain owing to a fractured ankle', 'rheumatoid arthritis', 'crying babies' and 'raised temperature'. Other research studies have looked at the value of Therapeutic Touch in relieving anxiety, post-operative pain, tension headaches, stress in newborn infants (who are, presumably, incapable of faith in the healing process) and in adults, and also its use in mental health nursing.

Professor Krieger went on to investigate whether it was necessary for a healer to be born with the ability or whether it might be taught. Eventually she proved that nurses could be trained to do healing but some were naturally better than others. Therapeutic Touch has caught the imagination of nurses in the USA and is now in mainstream practice. It has been slower to find favour in the UK and most other Western countries and many doctors and scientists appear to be unaware of the work that has been done.

In the course of researching this book, I have come across numerous examples of doctors and scientists – and a wide variety of self-appointed 'sceptics' – prepared to state categorically that there is no evidence that healing works. And if this condemnation before investigation is the case in the medical profession, what of the general population?

You may be one of those people who think that miracles are responsible for the results achieved by healers. You may believe that healing is just the operation of a natural science which we do not yet understand or that we have forgotten how to use. You may dismiss everything outside your knowledge or experience, or that you cannot easily and immediately comprehend, and decide that healing cannot work before reviewing any evidence. Alternatively, the whole idea of healing may offend some deeply held conviction or belief. Jesus is reported as saying, 'These things I do, so shall you do, and more.' This is not really open to much misinterpretation, but many Christians reject the idea that anyone other than Jesus could potentially be a healer of the mind, body and soul of others.

However, *beliefs* are not necessarily *truths*. And surely the best chance of arriving at truths is to consider the evidence with an open mind. So, whatever your initial position, I can only ask that you read the following brief introduction to healers and their work with an open mind.

HARRY EDWARDS & LORD LISTER/LOUIS PASTEUR

Harry Edwards was considered by many to be one of the world's greatest spiritual healers and was certainly an influential one. White-haired and stocky, in his smart dark suit he gave the impression of a city businessman. However, he was, by all accounts, something very different.

Harry was apparently guided by the spirits of Lord Lister, the founder of antiseptic surgery, and by Louis Pasteur, the famous French scientist. His patients ranged from the very poor to royalty, foreign rulers, cabinet ministers, army commanders, judges and bishops. Lady Baden-Powell, wife of the founder of the Boy Scout movement, was a regular visitor to his spiritual healing sanctuary at Shere, deep in the Surrey countryside. So too was Princess Marie Louise, grand-daughter of Queen Victoria. The famous conductor Sir Adrian Boult received healing from him, as did an ex-Queen of Spain.

Harry seemed to achieve miracles by soothing away pain, remoulding twisted limbs and restoring both sight and hearing. Sometimes he had results with what he called 'absent healing', when he was hundreds of miles away from the patient. He had absolutely no medical or surgical training.

Harry was born into humble surroundings in Islington in 1893 and began work as an apprentice in the publishing industry at the age of 14. In the First World War he served with the Royal Sussex Regiment and was promoted to acting major. Whilst stationed in Persia (now Iran) building railways and other projects he witnessed accidents and illness amongst his workers. His first aid kit consisted of little more than iodine, bandages and castor oil, but nevertheless he found that he was able to cure even the most terrible conditions by merely administering a mixture of first aid and quiet encouragement.

One day a local sheikh decided to bring his aged mother for treatment. Harry could see she was dying but dare not tell the sheikh. Instead, he prayed for guidance, prepared a potion from carbolic toothpowder and gave it to the woman. When the sheikh returned a few days later, with his guard of tribesmen shrieking and firing into the air, Edwards thought he was in big trouble. However, the old woman had completely recovered and the sheikh was bringing lavish gifts. Harry had to refuse them, but when pressed to accept something, said 'a few eggs' would be welcomed. Next day, 300 arrived!

After the war, Harry returned home, but maintained his interest in healing. His first contact with Spiritualism was at a church in Clements Road, Ilford. He was by no means an easy convert, but his psychic and healing powers soon began to develop more fully and in 1946 he bought a house at Shere in order to set up a healing centre. Within two years he was receiving around 3,500 letters a week and, as the number rose to over 9,000, he had to take on extra staff. His public demonstrations grew to fill the Royal Albert Hall.

Harry was instrumental in the formation of the National Federation of Spiritual Healers (NFSH) which now has over 7,000 members. The NFSH has long been developing and establishing a relationship with orthodox medicine and has been very successful. There is now a national doctor/healer referral network and many doctors have healers in their surgeries. In the light of their other activities, psychic surgery is still, perhaps, a little too controversial for the NFSH, however. Trance psychic surgery is explicitly forbidden in the NFSH Code of Conduct.

Harry Edwards continued healing until his passing on 7 December 1976. In his book, *Life in Spirit* (The Healer Publishing Co. Ltd, 1976), he outlines some of his thoughts on psychic surgery:

In this life, if we try to take one step out of our dimension of life, we cannot experience anything about it for it is 'not of this world'. A very wise doctor once appeared with the author on a television programme when films were shown of psychic surgery as practised in the Philippines. In these the Filipino healer was able to make an incision with his finger into the patient's body and to place his hand inside it, withdrawing a growth or some other fleshy substance. When the surgery was completed the healer would take his hands away from the body and the aperture was seen to be healed over without any sign of it having been opened at all ... The fleshy substance was available for inspection. After this the wound healed up as if by magic. There was not even a seam in the skin ... The doctor, observing this, said, 'I have seen this, but I cannot believe it, because if I did, it would be counter to all the knowledge and experience I have in medicine and surgery during my lifetime. I dare not accept it.'

The doctor's attitude is typical of so many. Betty Shine, the well-known author and healer, gives another example in her book *Mind Waves: The ultimate energy that could change the world* (Bantam Press, 1993):

There have been some incredible psychic surgeons. I was privileged to watch one of them performing an operation in London, during a public demonstration.
... I was standing beside a group of doctors who were talking amongst themselves. One of them remarked that if she had performed the same operation without anaesthetic, the patient would have been in agony. Nevertheless, they still did not believe what they had seen; I am sure they dismissed it as group hypnosis.

I have heard it said that some people are so attached to the 'Limitation Land' of their earthly experience that if a UFO full of aliens landed on their front lawn and a scouting party knocked on the door asking for directions, they would not believe it. If people really do limit their perceptions to this extent, it might prove impossible to convince them to broaden their horizons. Such people may, of course, have chosen this limitation at their higher self level, so that it is right for them to have this experience.

Here's the story of a woman whose experience was very different.

ROSE GLADDEN

Rose Gladden was only 19 when she walked into a dry-cleaning shop in London to find the owner slumped over the counter. He managed a cry for help: 'I have an ulcer.'

Rose had a strong desire to help him but had no idea what to do. A voice said, 'Put your hand there,' but she did not know where the problem was. Then she saw a tiny light, like a star, appear over his left shoulder and float down on to the right side of his stomach. She placed her hand on the light and then felt another unseen hand cover her own and hold it steady. A tremendous heat developed under her hand and she just could not pull it away. After a few seconds, the man recovered and told her the pain had gone. He rushed next door to tell people.

Rose had been born in Edmonton, London, in 1919 and had been having unusual experiences since she was seven years old. It now became clear that she was to use her talents for healing. She sought advice from another psychic and gradually developed her gift until she became one of the most dedicated and successful healers in Britain.

Early on, Rose saw everyone who turned up at her door. Later, she travelled thousands of miles on both sides of the Atlantic. In America and Canada, she lectured to medical specialists as well as to members of the public. She was asked by professors at several American universities to cooperate with them in tests and researchers at the University of California devised a system whereby she was wired up to a patient, a boy with a very serious nervous disorder, so that they could record what took place during the healing process. 'I am willing to submit to any test if it helps people to understand,' Rose said.

Maxwell Cade, a psychologist who has carried out pioneering work in meditation, relaxation and altered states of consciousness, also asked Rose to work with him. He reported finding distinctive brainwave patterns in healers. The research demonstrated that healers had a measurable effect on their patients, who after a few minutes picked up and imitated the same brainwave patterns. Rose Gladden was fascinated by this. For her it confirmed the importance of being 'attuned' to her patient.

As a natural psychic, Rose claimed to be able to see the aura, which she described as 'the protective circle of light and colour surrounding each human being'. She could apparently read the aura for ill health. One day she found she could also see silver spots and lines all over the surface of the body. It was not until some years later that she realized that these were the points and meridians used in acupuncture. People would describe their symptoms to her but she often felt their trouble was not where they thought it was. She often saw the 'real' trouble pinpointed by light. 'I'd put my hand in the light and the pain would go.'

As a sensible, practical woman, Rose was full of all sorts of advice. She once told a conference of nurses they must be sure to treat the dead with dignity as they often stayed with their discarded bodies for some time. She would also give patients advice on how to avoid repetition of their problem.

Rose knew that many doctors were not interested or even antagonistic towards her form of healing. She was, nevertheless, always quick to point out to her patients that healing is not a substitute for medicine, only a complement to it.

Chris Cole, a contemporary Australian healer and psychic surgeon, likewise comments: 'I always ask [my patients] if they have had a medical diagnosis.' She also says, 'It is not good for anyone to refuse orthodox treatment. Healing and psychic surgery are complementary, not alternative. The medical profession do a wonderful job but sometimes a different type of help is needed.'

Who could argue with that?

MATTHEW MANNING

One of the best known modern healers is Matthew Manning. From an early age he experienced voices, apparitions, objects (such as large metal beds) hurling themselves out of windows and a whole range of other psychic phenomena. He consented to all manner of scientific tests, but eventually tired of each new researcher – from countries as diverse as Sweden and Japan – wanting to conduct the same tests as others before them, because they just could not believe the results reported by their peers.

After a few unhappy years as a scientific and media curiosity, Matthew felt he should be doing something more positive with his unusual abilities. He left everything behind for a time, took a trip to India and made a pilgrimage to the Himalayas. It was there, looking out over the great mountains as the sun rose, that he started to realize that he had a capacity for healing and decided to devote his life to helping others. Thousands of people have benefited from his healing gift.

On television recently, when asked what he thought was behind the healing power, he simply said, 'Love.'

All genuine psychic surgeons seem to be agreed that the power of God, or love, works through them and that they are purely the instrument.

Such healers have been at work throughout history, but psychic surgery drew international attention in the 1960s with the work of a Brazilian, José Arigo.

JOSÉ ARIGO AND DR ADOLPHUS FRITZ

I saw him pick up what looked like a pair of nail scissors. He wiped them on his sports shirt and used no disinfectant of any kind. Then I saw him cut straight into the cornea of the patient's eye. She did not blench, although she was fully conscious. The cataract was out in a matter of seconds ... she was cured!

This was the remarkable testimony of Judge Immesi, witness to one of the many thousands of miracle cures performed by Brazilian psychic surgeon José Arigo – or rather Dr Adolphus Fritz, a German physician who, though dead since 1917, 'operated' directly through him.

Journalist Roy Stemman told *Psychic News* how it began. A priest had arrived to administer extreme unction to a dying woman:

Candles were lit and relatives and friends were gathered around her bedside in the town of Congonhas do Campo, Brazil. Her death, from cancer of the uterus, was expected at any moment. Suddenly, one of those present rushed from the room, returning moments later with a large knife from the kitchen. He ordered everyone to stand back. Then, without warning, he pulled the sheets from the woman and plunged the knife into her vagina. After several brutal twists of the blade he removed the knife and inserted his hand into the woman, withdrawing a huge tumour the size of a grapefruit. He dropped the knife and the bloody tumour in the kitchen sink, sat down on a chair and began to sob.

A relative rushed off to fetch a doctor; the rest stood silently as if transfixed ... The patient was unperturbed: she had felt no pain during the 'operation' and the doctor confirmed that no haemorrhaging or other ill-effects had occurred. He also confirmed that the growth in the kitchen sink was a uterine tumour.

... The man who performed the 'surgery', José Arigo, found himself in great demand ... yet he could not remember 'operating' on the woman.

Later, when such startling surgery became a daily occurrence ... it was realized that he was in a trance when he treated the sick...

On most days, when Arigo's clinic opened at 7 a.m., there was already a queue of 200 people waiting. Some he would treat in a rapid and often brutal fashion, pushing them against a wall, jabbing an unsterilized knife into them, then wiping it clean on his shirt. Yet they felt no pain or fear. There was very little blood, and the wound would knit together and heal within a matter of days.

Not everyone received psychic surgery. For many he would simply glance at them, diagnose their problems without any questions, then write a prescription rapidly. The medicines prescribed were usually well-known drugs made by leading companies, but in large doses and combinations that were surprising according to conventional medical doctors.

José Arigo died in 1971 and Stephen believes he has now joined his healing team. As he explained to *Psychic News* in 1987:

I saw clairvoyantly a man standing by my bed. The only words he spoke were, 'Surgeon with a rusty knife,' and he showed me the letter 'A'. When Dr

*Kahn was questioned he replied: 'There is a new
helper who has joined the healing band.'*

*None of this really made sense to me – until I
chanced to read an article about José Arigo. This
Brazilian healer, dubbed 'surgeon of the rusty knife',
was once jailed for 16 months for illegally practising
medicine. He used unsterilized scissors, knives or
scalpels – yet cured many thousands.*

Perhaps he is still curing many thousands ...

As for Dr Fritz, he moved on to using a practising medical
doctor as his instrument.

DR EDSON CAVALLIHO
AND DR ADOLPHUS FRITZ

Working in Brazil in the 1970s, Dr Edson Cavalliho, a fully
qualified obstetrician and gynaecologist, also practised deep-
trance psychic surgery with Dr Fritz. A documentary series,
The Psychic Connection, written, produced and directed by
Alan Neuman, shows the surgery which took place on a daily
basis whilst qualified radiologists, eye surgeons and patholo-
gists (on hand for the biopsies of tissues removed) looked on.

Dr Fritz seems to be enjoying himself on the film. He pro-
duces a foot-long hunting knife, removing it slowly from its
sheath in front of the next patient. The man seems a little
uneasy.

'I will use this *little* knife for demonstration purposes,'
the surgeon says with just a trace of a smile.

He runs the point of the knife approximately 8 inches (20
cm) down the man's spine. For a few seconds, nothing. Then, a
small amount of blood comes out as the wound opens up along
the length of the cut. The surgeon takes a surgical scalpel. He
motions for the sound man to bring the microphone nearer.

Viewers are treated to the squelching, gurgling sound of metal rotating, rubbing and scraping on flesh and bone. The patient seems oblivious. After removing the scalpel, Dr Fritz shows the flexibility of the wafer-thin instrument by breaking it between his finger and thumb. 'Look, it breaks easily,' he declares, 'but under the spiritual magnetic influence, it was as strong as wire cutters.'

Interviewed on the film about these events, Dr Lee Poulos, at the time assistant clinical professor at the Department of Psychiatry, University of British Colombia, offers an important reminder: 'I would warn against becoming totally enamoured with traditional, spiritual or psychic healing methods. Likewise modern medicine does not have all the answers. I would much prefer to suggest that each has its place.'

DONNA CICERA

Another healer working in Brazil in the 1970s was Donna Cicera, a Negro woman whom many believed to be a saint. Using an old pair of scissors and no antiseptic or anaesthetic, she would minister to two or three patients simultaneously. Then, after a day of healing, she would go home to begin looking after the 14 mentally and physically handicapped children who had been left on her doorstep at various times. She had adopted each of these children as her own.

Donna never refused anyone in need. Her clinic was paid for by donations. Flies were everywhere, dogs sauntered in and went to sleep under the operating tables, and patients who had been cured came back to help others. Donna could neither read nor write but nevertheless would perform complex, open-wound surgery on a daily basis. And it worked.

Donna's technique was to open very wide wounds in order to operate. She never sutured. Instead she would go into a deeper trance, put one hand either side of the incision and the two pieces of skin would come together. Then she would simply say, 'You can go now.' The wounds would only take a few days to heal instead of the more usual five or six weeks. Her trademark was a plastic tube. She used it in every operation, claiming that when she drew diseased material through it was when the real healing took place.

In another Alan Neuman documentary, Dr Beverly Morgan, a registered ophthalmological surgeon from California who had studied the healer's work, comments:

Donna would always insist that a prayer was read first by an assistant. She always behaved in a very reverent way. She explained to me that she heard a voice in her ear and this voice told her what was wrong. Someone said a team of doctors were helping her from another dimension. I watched her perform thoracic surgery, neuro-surgery, orthopaedic surgery and much more with the aid of this 'spiritual' guidance.

She told me: 'This is a very short incarnation for me. Make sure, if you are going to film, that you get good film.' One year to the day after saying this, she died of a cerebral aneurysm.

The most startling thing that struck me and others about Donna Cicera was her love and compassion for all who came her way.

As Alan Neuman himself added, 'Perhaps this is the lesson we can learn from her and others like her.'

LOURIVAL DE FREITAS

A South American healer practising in the 1960s was Lourival de Freitas. In the Christmas 1993 issue of *Psychic News*, journalist Tim Haigh recalled the visit of this famous psychic surgeon to Britain in July 1966:

> *This South American psychic astounded a 50 strong audience at the Spiritualist Association of Great Britain with some very graphic spirit surgery.*
>
> *PN's assistant editor of the time, Roy Stemman, felt his stomach turn over as he watched proceedings.*
>
> *'I had just seen a knife apparently plunged by [de Freitas] into the eye of a woman with a cataract,' he wrote.*
>
> *'I steeled myself and watched in astonishment as, after pressing on the eyelid, he squeezed a tiny object out into his hand. It was handed to a doctor, who identified it [as a cataract].'*
>
> *People may question the working practices of Stephen Turoff, but compared to de Freitas, they seem rather tame.*
>
> *Not only was the latter in full possession of his faculties, i.e. not entranced, but he was also in the habit of drinking generous quantities of whisky before beginning operations!*

As well as South America, the Philippines are known internationally for their healers. During my research, I have been fortunate to come into 'coincidental' contact with many people to whom I am indebted for their help, and one of these, Edna Drake from Canada, was kind enough to send me an article about a Filipino healer known to her simply as Benji, but to many others as Brother Benji Belacano.

BROTHER BENJI BELACANO

The article was written by an initially sceptical Western journalist called Clare Downs. She had a rare liver condition but was initially seeking an interview with Benji, not an operation:

Almost before I had time to become really terrified, Benji looked up and stated simply: 'We make an operation.' This was not what I wanted. I was about to speak out when I realized that something had entered my body. Benji's hand had penetrated my skin so easily that I could not conceive what was happening ... I held back. And just lay there. Terrified. Then it came to me. Faith healing – I must have faith ... At this point my intellect reminded me that I did not believe in God ...

I glanced down, and my worst fears were confirmed. Benji was drawing out a mass of tissue from around my liver. The tissue was deposited into a glass and the opening in my stomach was wiped down with a dampened piece of toilet paper. Finally Benji pressed gently but firmly on the opening and the next time I glanced down all that remained was a pinkish colour in the skin ...

Benji left soon after, saying that he would be back to perform another operation the next morning... During this operation I noticed Benji stuffing a lot of cotton wool inside me (at least I thought I saw it, I was too terrified to look down for too long). Next morning, after using the toilet, I looked down into the bowl and there was the cotton wool! Instantly I thought of the cynics, and wondered how they might explain this one.

Clare had studied both Latin and Greek and reported that Benji spoke both these languages fluently when under the control of different spirits. He apparently had no conscious knowledge of these languages. She and her colleagues also took convincing photographs of operations. Clare concludes: 'In Manila I saw things I thought I would never see, and felt things I had not conceived of. Only now can I see how limited were my visions of the world before.'

A brief review of psychic surgery around the world illustrates that it appears to be very different depending on the time and the place. This might have something to do with the target audience. As Dr Linda Chard says in her book *Dr Kahn: The Spirit Surgeon*:

The rural Filipino lives in a ... basic environment... His water probably comes from a lake within sight of his village.

Europeans and Americans are often far removed from the source of their amenities ... Science in Europe and America has reached the stage where its therapeutic and diagnostic equipment scans and treats with invisible rays and without touching the patient. Our minds can readily accept things which we do not see.

We are all advanced in some ways and vulnerable in others. The Spirit World chooses treatment appropriate to the cultural, mental and emotional background of each patient. A Westerner ... can accept ... unseen energies because his world already includes services provided by unseen sources. The Brazilian or Filipino would respond better if the diseased tissue were removed and laid aside for him to inspect. The Spirit World responds to the needs of each culture; psychic surgery in the Philippines is extremely physical whereas Western psychic surgery is less physical.

ALEX ORBITO

On the other side of the coin, Alex Orbito, a Filipino psychic surgeon says that it is Westerners who need to see the blood and other tissues in order to be convinced.

I interviewed Elisabeth Freeman, a nurse and naturopath from the United States, about her experiences with Alex. She told me that he used to visit healing centres and carry out demonstrations and healing sessions.

Orbito opened every day with a prayer and would break off at various times in the day to give little speeches about God's healing mission. He was never in full trance. If a patient asked a question, they could be sure that they were speaking to him rather than a spirit guide. His wife and one other helper generally assisted. Interestingly, Orbito's niece is also a psychic surgeon. Family members of healers may be more likely to become instruments themselves.

Elisabeth explained Orbito's technique:

Alex would enter the body with his fingers, at three points on the body. Initially there was a firm pressure on the skin and then suddenly the hands would slip inside. It didn't hurt. I had and watched many, many operations. Sometimes, large pieces of tissue would be removed. He explained that we Westerners

*needed to see in order to believe. The same result
could be achieved just by looking at the patient.*

Originally she went along to Alex:

*... with a hardened lymph node under my arm. After
one session, it had disappeared. A lump the size of a
Brazil nut had been removed in a few seconds. As a
nurse, I found this difficult to explain. But after a
while I decided I didn't need to explain, I needed to
believe.*

An interesting thought ...

Alex Orbito has spent time in jail for performing psychic
surgery in the US, where it is illegal.

JOSEPH MARTINEZ AND THE KAHUNAS

Elisabeth Freeman also told me about another Filipino who
works in the US. His name is Joseph Martinez and he performs 'mental psychic surgery'. This keeps him clear of any
threat of prosecution, as he does not touch the patient. When
people have treatment with him, they report that 'the room
fills with energy and you can feel the walls closing in around
you'. He apparently has 13 Kahunas – Hawaiian medicine men
– in his spirit team and it is they who perform the surgery
whilst the patient sits next to Martinez. Elisabeth says:

*Patients either give him their symptoms or they
don't. He doesn't mind either way. He is clairsen-
tient, which means that he feels the patient's problem in his own body. In some cases he tells the
patient to avoid stressing the area that has been
treated for up to six months, as this might affect the*

healing process. He also talks a great deal about magnetic healing and the forces that control the 'special magic' of psychic surgery.

Martinez has travelled all over the world. At one time, in Iran in the days of the Shah, he says he was kidnapped and taken to see a 'princess' who needed attention. It was made very clear to him that his surgery had better be successful!

Regarding 'magnetic healing', an interesting point is made by Richard Gerber, an American medical doctor who studied what he calls 'vibrational medicine' for 12 years before writing a book, *Vibrational Medicine* (Bear & Co., 1988), in which he explains:

An example of the lack of long-term benefit from magnetic types of healing can be seen with certain healings done by the 'psychic surgeons' of the Philippines. In some cases, cancer patients have returned with objective laboratory and clinical evidence of complete remission. However, some of these individuals have later returned to the same psychic surgeon several years later with a new tumour in a different organ system. Although a case may be made that the recurrent tumour was merely a metastic [secondary] lesion which was microscopic at the time of the original healing, there is a suggestion that the emotional/mental patterns of these patients which may have originally contributed to tumour formation were never addressed by the magnetic healer who worked primarily at the physical/etheric level.

Dr Gerber appears to be reiterating that dis-ease in the human body has its root in all levels of the self: physical, mental, emotional and spiritual. Dr Fritz holds a similar view – that illness develops on another plane of existence and filters down to the physical plane. True healing is achieved when all levels of self are treated simultaneously. Accordingly, to clear the physical level of the problem might leave it open to recurrence if the essential cause is not addressed at the original healing session. Many of the Filipino and other psychic surgeons do claim to be working at all levels, including the spiritual. Given this, they may not agree with Dr Gerber's interpretation.

However, it is not necessarily fair to say that the healer has 'failed' if full and total recovery is not achieved, especially if the patient goes back to old habits once the healer has tried to put right the results of previous bad habits.

The Brazilian and Filipino healers have generated a lot of publicity. Dr Kahn has said that, sometimes, influential people, like journalists and celebrities, are drawn to the healing work, often by their own or family health problems, in order that they might write or speak about it and thereby encourage others to try it for themselves.

An example of this can be found in the work of a British healer, George Chapman.

GEORGE CHAPMAN AND DR LANG

George Chapman was the healer that Kathy Turoff used to visit before she met Stephen. A former Aylesbury fireman, he claimed to be controlled by the spirit of William Lang, FRCS, late of the Middlesex and Moorfields Eye Hospital. Michael Chapman, George's son, is also a psychic surgeon.

Joe Bernard Hutton, a journalist threatened with blindness, was cured by George Chapman and went on to investigate further. He conducted many tape-recorded interviews with Dr Lang, both entranced and in his waking state. He cross-examined, stubbornly questioned and requested proof of any statement made. His findings are published in *Healing Hands: The amazing true story of a spirit doctor* (W. H. Allen, 1966; Virgin, 1995), in which he writes:

> *I travelled thousands of miles in Britain to interview those of Lang's patients I had picked out at random from Chapman's bulging case history files. As time went by, I had reel upon reel of tape-recorded statements from people who said that Lang had cured them. Some people claimed they had been cured completely by Lang, from diseases which hospital doctors had said were incurable.*
>
> *Apart from interviewing patients, I also checked their statements and medical histories. I wanted to be fully satisfied that I was in possession of facts and not highly coloured (and possibly inaccurate) emotional accounts.*
>
> *... I wish to make it abundantly clear that I have not the slightest intention of trying to influence or convert anyone to a new way of thinking, [merely to present] an objective account of the truth of the subject in question.*

What is Stephen's view of it all? He says simply:

> *My work is ... bringing people closer to God by showing them that what they think is science can be transcended by God whenever he chooses. Psychic surgery is spiritual science in action!*

7

PERSPECTIVES

Miracles do not happen in contradiction to nature, but only in contradiction to that which is known to us in nature.

ST AUGUSTINE

A wide variety of people have encountered Stephen Turoff. Their personal experiences are documented in various magazines, newspapers, books, videos, 'thank you' notes, clinic records and interviews. Some of their stories follow ...

THE ENERGY SCIENTIST

Energy is the ability of matter or radiation to do work.

Concise Oxford Dictionary

If the paranormal phenomena described throughout this book are 'real', then they can be measured. When we measure them they will become acceptable science, part of the natural order of things. What we currently lack are the instruments. This is not unusual in science. Before the microscope, many in the medical profession scoffed at the possibility of micro-organisms being the cause of unexplained deaths from operations.

In a sense then, nothing 'exists' until our Western scientific establishment says it does. In the meantime we are all scared to look foolish by going beyond the boundaries of what can be proven. One is labelled eccentric, misguided or even mentally unstable if one pursues these avenues of investigation seriously. Rational, analytical, brilliant minds who are prepared to cross the borders of orthodoxy and withstand peer pressure to search for truth are few and far between.

Fortunately, there are those in the world of science who retain a sense of awe and wonder at the enormity and beauty of God's many universes and are deeply spiritual in their search for knowledge. One such is Harry Oldfield, biologist by training, 'energy scientist' by experience.

Harry is a down-to-earth Christian who incorporates his spiritual outlook into both his research and the treatment of patients at his practice in Ruislip in northwest London. He invents instruments which are intended to help medical science gain a greater understanding of energy in relation to the human condition. An unintentional by-product of his work is the possibility of using his machines to investigate paranormal phenomena.

Harry's revolutionary research into 'energy medicine' has featured on the front covers of the *BMA News Review*, *Medical News Weekly*, the *Journal of Alternative & Complementary Medicine* and in the *Lancet* as well as in *The Times*, *Guardian*, *Independent* and *Daily Mail* newspapers. He has also made a number of television appearances and is co-author of *The Dark Side of the Brain* (Element, 1988).

Harry was at one time the world's leading researcher into Kirlian photography, a system of photographing the electrical activity of animate and inanimate objects which was discovered by accident in the 1930s when a Russian electrical engineer, Semyon Kirlian, chanced to pass his hand through an electro-magnetic field during experiments and saw a glow or 'corona' around it.

Harry used Kirlian photography to show that the electrical energy of a whole leaf was still present when most of the physical leaf had been cut away and discarded. This appeared to indicate that the energy body was a *blueprint* onto which physical molecules were attached. He showed how certain natural, organic foods (e.g. muesli) had a lot of electrical energy, whereas processed foods (e.g. cornflakes) had none. In experiments at major London hospitals, such as Charing Cross, he then noticed that certain diseases created larger than average coronas in Kirlian pictures of patients (e.g. cancer) whilst others created smaller than average coronas (e.g. arthritis). This led on to the design of instruments and machines for the diagnosis and treatment of the energy field of sick people.

In 1981, the *Guardian* reported, in its science section, that Harry had measured and recorded what he called 'seven energy-configuration points' around the body. This led him in to a whole new area. In traditional healing theory, the body has 'energy channels' (meridians), 'energy whirlpools' (chakras) and 'auric colours' which have been used as the basis for diagnosis and treatment for thousands of years. Modern Western science has been largely dismissive of this 'mumbo-jumbo'. Had Harry stumbled on a way of scientifically measuring these channels, whirlpools and colours in the energy field? Much of the subsequent evidence suggested that this was indeed the case.

Whilst on a lecture tour in the USA, Harry met Richard Gerber, the author of *Vibrational Medicine*. Dr Gerber suggested that he try using the emerging computer technology to devise an energy field scanner which could actually show the field in full moving colour. Today Harry uses what he has called polycontrast interface photography (PIP) to display a person's energy field on a computer screen.

Stephen Turoff sees the colours, channels and whirlpools of the energy field with his own eyes, so early in 1995 we invited him to meet Harry for research purposes and an exchange of ideas. Present at the research session were myself, Jane, Harry Oldfield and Len Randall, a man with an interest in all things metaphysical and paranormal. What we witnessed was truly amazing and I am still struggling to believe it actually happened.

In Harry's 'PIP studio', where he has set up his energy field photography equipment, Stephen stood against the white background which hangs from the ceiling to the floor. Harry manned the video camera and asked me to be in charge of the computer mouse. Jane and Len were to watch Stephen and the computer screen for anything unusual.

Stephen put his head back slightly and began concentrating, putting himself in what he calls 'healing mode'. After very few seconds, a circle of yellow light appeared above his head on the computer screen. It changed colour to pink and then white.

'We may be witnessing a portal to another dimension,' mused Harry excitedly.

'I haven't really started concentrating yet,' said Stephen, grinning.

Just then, Harry shouted at me, 'Quick! Grab it! There's a face on the screen!'

All eyes surveyed the screen. A face was forming, as if coming through into the circle from behind the screen. It was a man's face. He had a beard. It looked like Dr Kahn. He smiled! A cheeky grin. Then he disappeared.

I had clicked the mouse at just the right moment and caught the circle of white light on the screen. But when we printed it out, there was no face, just the light. (The picture is now on display at the Danbury Healing Clinic.) Although disappointed not to have a picture to show the inevitable army of sceptics, all five people in that room knew that a major first had just occurred: the face of a person from another dimension of reality, another world, had been seen with modern technology. This meant that it could be repeated in the future. We were all very excited. Just as the first microscope helped people see tiny organisms from the 'micro-universe', so we might now have a machine to help us see the 'energy-universe'.

I have already suggested that other worlds could occupy the same space as ours, but operate on much higher vibrations or frequencies. Is it feasible that, if it was Dr Kahn on the screen, he might have lowered his own vibration or operating frequency to precisely the right one to be picked up by Harry's machine?

Stephen had also brought with him some of the sacred ash, or *vibhuti*, which had formed on the pictures at his clinic. The ash was put into a small brown open-topped envelope and photographed with Len Randall holding it. This PIP picture shows energy, represented by pink and gold light, emanating from the supposedly dead ash. Other researchers have apparently found that this ash contains substances that cannot be found anywhere else on the planet.

Another aspect of Harry's work is the development of what he calls 'electro-crystal therapy'. Harry is an acknowledged scientific expert on the properties of crystals, which he claims have a variety of therapeutic uses:

> *Crystals cause changes in brainwave patterns which can be measured on EEG monitors. If you hold a crystal in your hand the frequency of your own macro-molecules, which resonate a complex waveform, can imprint itself into the otherwise regular oscillations of the crystal lattice. So, the crystal's electrons will move in regular fashion vibrating exactly like your own macro-molecules. The crystal appears to copy your own specific wave-form.*

If you heat a crystal you get electrical energy. If you squeeze it you get light. If you introduce a certain impurity you get a particular visible wavelength (colour). Subtle changes in the coating of a crystal can be used to detect very small changes in frequency caused by linking an antibody to a specific pesticide like malathion. Crystals can be placed over meters in houses to regulate pollution from 'negative' energies. Crystals are even used to measure changes in radio wavelengths and can receive and amplify complicated wave-forms emanating from radio-transmitters hundreds of miles away. Given these phenomena, it should come of no surprise that crystals are very sensitive indeed to the subtlest of energies.

Crystals can also work in reverse, themselves amplifying specific harmonics; and in this lies the basis of electro-crystal therapy. Given the premise that disease is caused by a cell or group of cells going 'out of tune', then the action of a crystal is to receive the correct 'healthy' signal and rebroadcast it, so that the specific 'normal' wavelength can be pushed back into the cell and thus carry out a retuning function.

Given research such as this, it seems that there are many exciting new medical breakthroughs to come. And just recently, there has been a new development in psychic surgery. In the summer '96 issue of *Kindred Spirit*, journalist Chris Stoner asked Stephen about it:

Stephen clears his throat. 'During the last year there have been a number of examples where patients have received new organs. The team are able to create them in their world and manifest the organ into the physical. God alone knows how they do it.'

... In an attempt to shed some light on the matter, I first visit Robin Foy, founder of the Scole-based New Spiritual Science Foundation.

'During the last few years a new energy, resonating at a higher vibratory rate, has been beamed down to Earth. This has greatly helped the Spirit world to work more closely with us. Through the group's physical mediumship we have already seen over 100 different phenomena – at least one third of which are brand new. The techniques used to materialize these, and other, objects are also very different. Ectoplasm is now a thing of the past.'

Robin believes that, as this new energy increases, a gateway between the two dimensions will occur. Communication between us and the dead will become a normal, everyday happening.

Stephen also believes that this will be the future and that those unable to communicate 'naturally' will be able to do so via machines.

THE SPIRITUALIST CHURCH OF SANDVIKEN, SWEDEN

In 1991, a detailed account was written by the Spiritualist church of Sandviken of Stephen and Kathy's visit there. This gives an idea of what may happen at a psychic healing demonstration.

First, Dr Gino, an Italian spirit doctor, came through and spoke to the audience. He treated a 14-year-old boy who was mentally retarded. (We can speculate that this is his speciality although nothing was said to this effect.)

Then Dr Kahn came through as usual. The first patient – the report used assumed names – was Lotta from Gavle.

Stephen was assisted by Kathy and two church officers. Following a prayer, Dr Kahn examined his patient. The spirit surgeon explained he would perform an operation on her abdomen, saying also that an injection would be necessary. Though the hypodermic syringe was not visible, a small hole appeared. The report continued:

> After that, Dr Kahn took a piece of cotton wool, which he dipped into a bowl of water. All of us then saw his hands, as far as the knuckles, disappear into Lotta's stomach. From the movements of Dr Kahn's hands, we understood he was cleaning it. [Removing his hands,] the piece of cotton wool was dripping with fluid. Later, some red marks appeared on the patient's abdomen.
>
> After some minutes, these faded and totally disappeared. Dr Kahn said he would now perform a spiritual operation on one of Lotta's ovaries, since something was wrong with it. Small dark red blood clots appeared. Though a small scar was visible, it vanished after three days.

Later, Lotta said that whilst she felt Dr Kahn's hands inside her body, it had not been painful. 'Only the spiritual hypodermic syringe ... felt a little tender.'

Another patient, Ingrid, who had injured her knees over 30 years previously, said that before Stephen's visit to Sweden, she had received a message from her spirit guide that a man named Joseph could help make her well. One night she saw three spirit doctors standing around her bed. Ingrid also noticed a man with a black beard who held up a piece of cloth with the initials 'J. K.'. Later, in a Swedish magazine called *Utan Grans*, she saw a picture of Dr Joseph Kahn, who was identical to the man with the black beard. She immediately called the Spiritualist Association and arranged for an operation. According to the report:

> *When she finally met Dr Kahn he told her he had visited her before, at night. During treatment Dr Kahn straightened out Ingrid's badly twisted spine, noting that she had a blood condition. Ingrid felt good after the operation. The pain totally disappeared from her knees.*

The third patient was a woman called Rut who sought help for a heart condition. This was a rare problem, inherited from her mother's side of the family. Doctors had explained that they could do nothing for her. Dr Kahn told Rut there was nothing wrong with her heart, but he detected a congenital blockage in the aorta. The spirit surgeon 'removed the blockage by dematerializing some small black-red blood cells from the aorta. He told her to take these clots with her and have them analysed in hospital, to be confirmed it really was her own blood.'

Another Swedish woman who was tested in hospital after psychic surgery was Lena, a patient with an ulcerated colon. She had earlier been admitted to hospital but had refused permission for the entire colon to be removed. After an operation by Dr Kahn, she returned to hospital and underwent a blood test. Though the doctors were expecting the blood count to have dropped, 'to their great surprise' it had increased.

THE ISRAELIS

In March 1993, a large group of people came over from Israel, following coverage of Stephen's work there. As a result of the success of this trip, they invited Stephen to visit their country. On Monday 28 June 1993, Stephen and Kathy travelled to

Israel for one week. They stayed in a traditional Israeli house and were made very welcome. One family brought a man in a wheelchair. He had suffered a major stroke. The hospital could do no more for him. He could not move or speak. He had to be spoon-fed. Dr Kahn saw him over a period of five days for about five minutes each day. At the end of the week he was talking and laughing and could feed himself.

Stephen now regularly visits Israel about four times a year. Because of the number of people treated in each session, the spirit team 'up the energy'. 'God has no limitation,' says Dr Kahn. The power used is so great that some patients receive just a blow of breath and a tap on the problem area. People have got up out of wheelchairs and walked home following this treatment.

THE CHILDMINDER

Jane and I had been giving hands-on healing to Ann Bradford, a friend of my mother's who always has a house full of children. (She used to look after me when I was young, poor woman.) Unfortunately, she had suffered with cancer for a while and we suggested an appointment with Stephen. She looked at us rather sheepishly and said, 'I hope you don't mind, but a friend of mine has arranged to see him and she booked me in at the same time. I'm going next week.'

Later, she told us what happened:

I went with my daughter-in-law Helen and her friend, who had a clot of blood on her lung. When we arrived we sat in the waiting room for a while. There was a video playing. I'm a Christian but it was lovely to see all the many different people and religions represented at the clinic. We watched the video which showed Sai Baba walking amongst the crowds and then we went for a cup of coffee in the hotel. We listened as people around us chatted excitedly about their experiences. What they were saying was a bit difficult to take in. It didn't put me off though ...

'Sorry about the wait,' Stephen said when we went in to the small room. He didn't say anything else until my daughter-in-law's friend was on the table. He pointed his finger at her and asked, 'What do you expect me to do for you when you are abusing your body?' Helen and I sat in the corner looking at the floor.

When my turn came I told him I had breast cancer. He put his hands flat on my lungs. Then he pulled up my jumper and picked up a scalpel. I remember thinking, Ow! He's cut me, but it didn't hurt. It was as if I had been given a local anaesthetic. Then he flopped something into the bucket. I heard it drop. I had my eyes closed but could feel the blood running all over me. Then he used swabs to mop it all up. All I could think about was the mess the blood would make on my white jumper. He placed one hand on my body and the other on my forehead and, looking up to the ceiling, he began muttering a chant, over and over again. I opened my eyes and he stared into them. His eyes were like deep blue pools.

'Do try to come back to see me. I need to see you again. Please try.' He left the room.

I walked out of the room and thought, That's it, I'm cured. Then I saw the notice on the wall: 'Stephen Turoff is a healer, not a doctor. Do not stop your medication unless advised by your own doctor.' This seemed like good advice. On the way home, and for the next few days, it was as if I was on a high.

I could not stop talking about my experience. I booked another appointment.

The next time Stephen was much more chatty. Whilst he was laying his hands on me he began talking to Helen as if he knew her.

'How is your back?' he asked. She had never had any treatment from him before and was surprised that he knew about her back.

'I've been in a lot of pain.'

'I know, your kidney stone has returned. Take olive oil and lemon juice, a tablespoon of it, for three days,' he advised. 'I'm going in here,' he said, suddenly changing his tone of voice. He cut me open. Helen told me later that his hands disappeared into my body. He gave me an injection. It was a proper syringe – but it didn't have a needle! I felt the liquid going in. He swabbed up the mess as before and pressed the cut together. Then he put his hands on my body and on my head as before. When I sat up, a grey ash was in my hair. He smiled and left. He didn't tell me to come back, I thought. I waited to speak to him. I caught him as he moved between the operating rooms.

'You are doing so well,' he said, 'if you would like to come back then I shall be pleased to see you.' But I have decided not to go back because I don't feel the need. I feel in my heart that I am cured.

A few days before we saw her for this interview, Ann had been for a bone scan. It was clear. We were just leaving when she remembered another story and said excitedly:

I must tell you about a friend of mine who went to see Stephen. She was depressed and had a number of things wrong.

'There's nothing wrong with you at all,' she was told by Stephen. 'If you don't stop worrying, and having all this stress, you will have a heart attack. The past is gone, the future is uncertain, now is the moment in which to live.'

My friend was unconvinced. Then, as she was going out the door, he said something that stopped her in her tracks. 'Who is this man I have here? He tells me that Stanley is his name. And another man is here, too. He is pointing to his ring and saying, "Ring, ring, ring." Does this mean anything to you?'

My friend realized that Stephen must be able to see her father and her husband, who have both passed on. No one could have known what that ring meant to her. It was between her and her husband. She had no other explanation than that they must both be there, watching over her. This was a great comfort. She left much happier.

THE DISSATISFIED PATIENTS

The majority of patients who visit the Danbury Healing Clinic do feel better for their experience, but there are people who go away unhappy. One lady went to Stephen with cancer. The tumours were numerous, hard and large.

'You silly woman,' admonished Dr Kahn, 'why have you not been to the hospital?'

The lady in question was scared of hospitals and had refused the normal orthodox treatment. She was not at all pleased to be talked to like this.

'Don't you tell me what to do!' she retorted. 'It's my body and I'll do what I please.'

This, of course, was her prerogative and Dr Kahn left it at that.

Others who sometimes react badly to Dr Kahn's scolding are those whose smoking, drinking or other habits have caused or contributed to their problems.

Dr Kahn tells us that he was by no means a saint himself when he lived on Earth. But when people come asking for healing, he can only do so much for them. It is they themselves who are the architects of their own dis-ease ('distance' from the 'ease' that is oneness with God). And it is only through *change* that progress towards health will be achieved. Change in physical, mental, emotional and spiritual 'well-being' will only be achieved by change in physical, mental, emotional and spiritual 'ways of being'.

Having said this, Dr Kahn and Stephen are very effective in the way that they put this message across. This may be one reason why, of every hundred patients seen, only about five have what they consider to be an unsatisfactory experience.

THE NOAH'S ARK SOCIETY

At the end of January 1993, Stephen and Dr Kahn demonstrated for the Noah's Ark Society during a residential week at the Arthur Findlay College, Stansted Hall, Essex. The Society's purpose is to investigate metaphysical and paranormal phenomena.

Public and private treatments were given for a variety of ailments. In front of over 100 people Dr Kahn appeared to remove a tumour from a woman he said had a growth on her liver. A man who suffered back pain seemed to have a piece of bone removed from his spine. During this psychic operation, Dr Kahn claimed that he was one of a team of 18 spirit beings present.

A woman worried about whether a conventional heart operation had been successful was diagnosed as having infected lungs. Dr Kahn told her that she would no longer be in this world in six to 10 months if she continued to smoke. Two pairs of surgical scissors were used to treat her chest and could be seen sticking out of it, yet she said she felt no pain. Observers were invited on to the platform to witness the wound heal up.

A psychic operation on a back sufferer who claimed to have a crushed vertebra resulted in the most startling treatment of the afternoon. According to the Society's report of the proceedings, Dr Kahn

> ... appeared to make a small incision with a scalpel approximately six inches [15 cm] up from the base of the spine. A small cut appeared. Next to it he placed a five pence piece on which he lit some gauze. Covering it with a small glass and then a towel, he stood back and explained that he was attempting to draw out a blood clot, which, he maintained, would turn into a tumour if not removed. After some three to four minutes the towel was taken away and the glass appeared to be full of blood.

A blood clot about an inch in diameter was 'clearly evident'. Dr Kahn explained that the vacuum created in the glass – due to the burning gauze using up all the air inside – had drawn the clot up the spinal track. He insisted the patient take it away to be analysed.

A woman claiming to be suffering from fibroids of the womb came in for treatment and said she'd 'love to have a hysterectomy'. Dr Kahn decided to operate. He told the patient he was going to give her an injection and, reaching from behind, seemed to take hold of an invisible syringe. The woman stated that she could feel the needle going in. Then Dr Kahn placed his hand over her face and told her to take deep breaths.

Elizabeth Wheeler, general secretary of the Noah's Ark Society, who was holding the patient's head, was also asked to breathe into the spirit surgeon's hand. Later, she described feeling 'exceptionally tranquil' as a result. The spirit doctor began treatment on the patient's stomach using various instruments. When asked to explain how this procedure benefited the patient, he said simply, 'It is a matter of altering the structure of the cells.'

THE MOTHER AND DAUGHTER FROM CYPRUS

When they went to see Stephen in 1987, Semra Karahassan, from Cyprus, and her daughter, Paula, then 25, were left in no doubt about Stephen's power. Semra believes that Stephen cured her of cervical cancer.

'When I met him I thought he couldn't possibly do miracles,' she said. 'He was far too ordinary and jokey.' But when she lay on the operating bed, with Paula at her side, what happened was far from ordinary.

First they saw the change in Stephen's voice and appearance. Then, after administering a psychic injection which made Semra drowsy, Dr Kahn picked up a scalpel and made an incision.

I was so scared, I went, 'Ow, it hurts!' And he said in his German accent, 'My good woman, I can assure you, you are feeling no pain.' And he was right – it didn't hurt at all. I was just panicking. He put in his fingers to open the cut wider, and then, using an instrument, he pulled out something muscley, about as big as a whole nut, with blood on it.

As soon as they arrived home, Semra and Paula examined the cut and found the red scar almost healed. Semra had been booked into hospital for an exploratory operation. By the time she attended, the scar had vanished. Semra was sure that Stephen Turoff was not putting on an act or using a magic trick. 'He didn't charge me,' she says. 'Why would he go to all that bother if it wasn't to make money? I know it's extraordinary, but I promise it all happened.'

THE SWISS JOURNALIST

Jaime T. Licauco is a Swiss journalist with an interest in psychic surgery. He flew from Zurich to London to witness Stephen's healing, but ended up having it done to himself:

I'd seen Brazilian psychic surgeons, such as José Arigo, perform gruesome and bloody psychic operations on patients with their crude instruments (e.g. blunt knives, scissors, etc.) on videotape before and once in person in Sao Paulo, Brazil. I couldn't stand the sight of them. I never for once ever dreamed that I would experience such a surgery performed on myself, but that was exactly what happened to me in London in October 1990. A five-inch [12 cm] steel knife was fully inserted inside my right nostril.

We [had] asked Stephen Turoff if we could witness him go into a trance and talk to Dr Kahn ... In a few minutes he was in a trance, his eyes staring blankly. We asked who he was and received the reply: 'My name is Pafi. I am an Egyptian who left your world in 1950. This is only the second time I am coming through this instrument' (meaning Stephen). Pafi said he was also a healer and pointed to me as having a problem with my nose. This was true. Pafi said I had a nodule inside my nose which he would take out.

Thereupon, he announced, 'I need a knife.'

... He rejected the first ones brought to him from the kitchen as too wide. He needed a knife with a thin blade, he said. Shortly afterwards, somebody produced a thin-bladed knife, about five inches long. 'This will do,' he announced mechanically.

... I really got scared ... but on the other hand, I was curious. Pafi (Stephen) motioned for me to lie on the table ... Soon I felt a strong discomfort as the whole blade was inserted inside my right nostril. I groaned and moaned in pain, but it was not an ordinary pain I felt. It was more of a discomfort at having a long, sharp piece of steel inside my nose. I wanted him to take the knife out but he seemed to be taking his sweet time and even twisted the knife inside my nose.

Pafi said there was really no pain but the reason I was groaning was that I had a low threshold of pain and that my fears had made my muscles tense, which was true. I was really tense and who wouldn't be under those circumstances! The video cameras, meanwhile, recorded my whole ordeal.

After a while he removed the knife and out came phlegm and some blood. He then asked me to blow my nose on a tissue paper, which I did. More phlegm came out. My breathing cleared up. I got up off the table and thanked him for the healing. I saw everybody staring at me. I said I was all right.

THE PSYCHIC NEWS EDITOR

In their 6 February 1993 issue, *Psychic News* made a statement of the newspaper's official position with regard to Stephen's psychic surgery:

Stephen Turoff is perhaps the most controversial healer working today. Understandably his methods have provoked mixed reactions over the years ...

Having witnessed Stephen's work at close hand, PN believes his trance state to be genuine. PN also concludes that his healing technique, although somewhat disturbing to watch at times, presents no risk to patients.

The paper's view is based on testimony from those who have had psychic operations at the hands of Dr Kahn, from experienced healers who have witnessed Stephen's work, and from seeing with our own eyes what takes place in the course of a consultation.

However, the lack of medical evidence that 'cures' have taken place must be noted. Until such a time as it is presented, PN is not in a position to comment on the efficacy of Stephen's healing.

However, statements from sufferers commenting they no longer feel pain or discomfort after treatment – and PN has many on record – serve as testimony to Stephen's gifts and cannot be ignored.

THE SONGWRITER

Sonya Madan is singer and lyricist with the rock group Echobelly. While touring America she found a copy of *Kindred Spirit* magazine on the floor of a bus. There was an article in it on electro-crystal therapy and Sonya resolved to try Harry Oldfield's clinic when next in London. She had already heard of Stephen:

> *I first heard about Stephen Turoff from a friend who had met a woman at a dinner party who claimed that a psychic surgeon had cured a problem in one of her eyes and stopped her from going blind. We managed to trace Stephen's number and I made an appointment myself.*
>
> *I had started healing sessions at Harry Oldfield's clinic and it was there that I picked up another copy of the magazine* Kindred Spirit *which happened to have an article on Stephen. As I was a relative newcomer to alternative healing, the article helped explain what I should expect and gave an insight into this strange phenomenon.*
>
> *When the day of the appointment came, I was quite excited and also a bit nervous at the thought of being 'operated' on in this way. I'd been ill for about two years with a hyperactive thyroid and had also developed polycystic ovaries. I'd been on medication but the only 'cures' offered were a drastic operation or a radioactive iodine drink.*
>
> *I sat in the waiting room with a lot of other people. There were pictures of Jesus and Sai Baba, there were written messages on the walls and an ash-like substance growing on some of the pictures. I felt really comfortable there and it was only when it was*

my turn to be taken into the healing room and I saw
the scissors and scalpels that I started to think about
where I was.

When Stephen Turoff came into the room, he
appeared abrupt and in a bit of a hurry. He asked
what was wrong, loosened my jeans and put a cloth
on my stomach and picked up a pair of scissors.

My sister, who had accompanied me, was sitting
in a corner of the room. She looked pretty scared
when she saw the scissors. It all happened very quickly. It was the strangest thing to hear the sound of
flesh being cut and to feel cold metal instruments
moving inside me, but there was no pain, it was just
a bit uncomfortable.

I remember saying, 'God, you don't waste any
time,' and Stephen replied (in an interesting accent),
'Why should I waste time, I have a coachload of
Welsh people coming later.'

He put his hand on my stomach and then pulled
something out of me, rubbed some ash on the area
and just as quickly started on my throat. He said,
'You are a writer,' more as a statement than a question. I remember mumbling something but not being
able to talk for the surprise of what was happening.

It wasn't until Stephen put a hand on my forehead that I began to relax and I felt very peaceful
when this happened, almost elated. There were questions I wanted to ask but there didn't seem to be any
time. It was all over.

On the way home I kept looking at the areas
where the cuts had been made. There were two
puncture marks and a jagged semi-circle and the
smell of incense. The marks disappeared after a few
days, but I'll never forget that day and I am very

grateful to Stephen Turoff for helping me. I have had
some tests since and I am perfectly fine.

THE WAR VETERAN FROM BROADSTAIRS

Ben Tillott is a veteran of the Second World War. His problem
started during August 1992, during a reunion to celebrate the
liberation of Arras, in France. Mr Tillott was required to
sound the *Last Post* and *Reveille* at various cemeteries and
memorials. He started getting pains down both legs and it was
becoming very difficult to walk. He managed to complete his
tasks and returned home thinking that the problem was tem-
porary, but this was not the case.

A few weeks later he went to see his doctor, who sent
him for X-rays. He was told a week later that he had arthritis
in the hip, but he was dubious as to the accuracy of this
diagnosis and received no benefit from the prescribed pain-
killers. Then came an appointment with a neurologist – for
three months hence. In the meantime Mr Tillott was visiting an orthopaedic specialist. After 12 25-minute sessions
he felt little benefit. By January 1993 the pain was so bad
that he asked his doctor for a private appointment with the
neurologist.

Some time later, he became a patient at the Royal Sea
Bathing Hospital at Margate for a three-week course of therapy in the gym and pool. Once again there was no improvement. He then attended Thanet General Hospital three times
a week for continued therapy. After four weeks there was no
improvement.

He had the private appointment with the neurologist and
the X-rays showed a protrusion on the fourth lumbar vertebra,
which the neurologist thought might be a disc problem. By
now Mr Tillott was also visiting a chiropractor and, after
showing him the X-rays, was told that the problem was a bone

protrusion. This treatment gave some relief from pain but did not offer a cure.

The neurologist sent him to Canterbury Hospital for a scan. This gave no more information about the spine but indicated a swollen aorta. He now had to visit a cardiac specialist at Margate who confirmed the aorta condition but was positive it had no bearing on the leg pain, which was a 'nerve problem'. When he requested the removal of the bone protrusion he was told that this would be difficult and dangerous.

The day after seeing the cardiac specialist, Mr Tillott visited the Danbury Healing Clinic. It was now August 1993, a year after the symptoms first manifested. Mr Tillott explains:

For the whole of that year I had been using two elbow crutches or two walking sticks ... At Danbury, I literally hobbled into the clinic on two sticks, with the pains right down both legs and my feet quite numb and tingling, as they had been for the past year, continuously.

Dr Kahn saw me and after a chat about my condition, massaged my aorta and then took away the protrusion on my lumbar.

I walked out of the consulting room without using the two sticks and have not used them since! I am now doing things that I have not been able to do for more than a year – cutting the grass, riding my motorcycle, going for quite long walks, turning over in bed without having to sit up.

I was able to visit Arras again and take part in the weekend activities absolutely free from any sign of pain or ache.

I shall be eternally grateful to Dr Kahn for returning me to a normal lifestyle.

THE SURPRISED PHOTOGRAPHER

The following is a letter from a lady who tried to take a photograph at the clinic.

Dear Grant,

Here are the details of our visit to Stephen's on Friday 29th November [1996].

My friend Veronica was being treated by Stephen for arthritis of the hands for the first time and I was in the room looking on. We asked Stephen whether he minded if we took some photographs ... He said: 'Yes, of course, go ahead.' I took two photographs of Stephen working, perfectly normal, no problem.

It was then my turn to get up onto the bed as I had problems with my legs and back. Stephen was working on my legs and I must admit I was feeling extremely hot, so hot in fact that my glasses steamed up! I actually asked Stephen whether this heat was coming from him and he just blew out some air in my direction, smiled, winked and carried on working without saying a thing. My friend Veronica was trying to take a photograph of me at this point and the camera just wouldn't work, no matter what she did. Stephen said it probably needed the photograph of 'Baba' to help so he took the photograph off the wall and placed it beside my legs. Still no picture, so he told my friend to pass the camera to me to see if I could get it to work. I couldn't get it to work either.

By this time we were all joking about it. Stephen looked up to the ceiling and said, 'What on Earth have you sent me today? What a pair.' He then asked for the camera and said, 'Let's see what I can do.' Stephen did everything to try to get the camera to work, only to have the shutters shut and not open up either, so he said, 'I think the camera has had it, it won't do anything at all now!' He carried on with my other leg.

When Veronica and I got outside in the car, I asked her what her stomach looked like after the operation. Well, she had a scar so we thought we would see if the camera would work. I took it out of the case and put my finger on the shutter button, whereupon the camera took a picture without me going near the proper button ... If I had not have been with my friend to witness the fact that I didn't touch this button, nobody would have believed us.

I haven't had the pictures developed yet but we went on to take some of the outside of the building without any problems whatsoever.

We went to Stephen with a completely open mind and came away spiritually uplifted, healed, amazed and truly thankful for everything he does, not only for us but for everyone who turns to him.

Cathy Acres and Veronica Cain
Surrey

This may seem like a case of faulty photographic equipment. However, so many strange phenomena are reported in connection with cameras and photographs at Stephen's clinic that it is very difficult not to believe that something is influencing the photography.

THE CLAIRVOYANT

Joan Green is a clairvoyant who lives in Reading. Her husband, George, is a healer. They were the couple who first introduced Esteban Molina to Stephen. Prior to her visit to see Stephen, Joan had been conducting a reading for a client.

'I have a German spirit doctor with you,' she said. 'I don't know why he is here.'

'I am checking up on my patient!' communicated the German doctor sternly.

'Well,' explained Joan, 'you can imagine what I thought about this rather abrupt spirit person. Arrogant little German, I thought to myself and then forgot about it.'

Then, when she went to the clinic:

We walked in to see Stephen, who was already entranced by his guide. You can imagine my shock when he looked up at me, grinned and said, 'Ach so! An arrogant little German, am I?'

I didn't know where to put myself. Dr Kahn had read my rude thoughts and here I was next in line for a psychic operation. Luckily he has a great sense of humour and was more amused than upset. We got along fine. He operated on my knee and it worked.

Finally, here are some more personal perspectives...

JASON – THE SON'S PERSPECTIVE

Jason Turoff goes to work sporting a smart suit and silk tie, with his long hair tied back in a neat pony tail. He is a fit, strong and healthy young man. Like his father, he stands well over six feet tall. He appears to have the patience of a saint. These are useful attributes for one of his least favourite jobs – when called upon, he is the bouncer at the Danbury Healing Clinic! Believe it or not, people push and shove and even fight to get in to see Stephen before someone else.

Frayed tempers might sometimes be due to the long wait. It might be that an ambulance turns up and the patient inside is treated 'out of turn'. At other times people refuse to pay, or try to leave without paying. It might be that someone tries to jump the queue. Sometimes a whole coachload of people turns up without booking.

Mostly, of course, there is just the routine problem of organizing large groups of sick people and their friends and relatives in a confined space. They shout and complain. They lock themselves in the toilet. People will be people!

Most days, there is no let up in the constant stream of people wanting Jason's attention. From dealing with the crowd, who are often waiting outside the closed clinic as he arrives, to tidying up when everyone has left, Jason is called upon to deal calmly and politely with anything and everything. Despite all these problems, he enjoys his work. His father has encouraged him to start healing, but he is not yet sure if he wants to go down that path.

KATHY – THE WIFE'S PERSPECTIVE

The following is from an interview I conducted with Kathy in July 1996.

'How did you feel about Stephen's work at first?'

'I was very interested in helping. It is a good feeling to be able to help people like this.'

'What did you think when Dr Kahn first came through in 1985?'

'Well, as you can imagine, I thought I'd seen it all by then. What with things moving in the house, transfiguration demonstrations and everything else, I didn't think it could get much more unusual.'

'What could you say to other healers who are considering going full time?'

'We wouldn't have survived without my income. Then, as the talks and demonstrations built up, so did the number of people coming. We know now that the spirit team needed time to get everything ready before the hoards of people could be coped with, but that's hindsight. When Stephen wasn't very busy, we had serious doubts about whether it was going to work.

'If I had one thing to say to a healer who was going to go full time it would be: "Make sure your partner is 100 per cent behind you. Take good account of the fact that you need to live, pay the bills and eat."

'I know that sounds a bit simplistic, but there have been quite a few healers who have gone full time expecting it to just happen overnight. This certainly wasn't the case with us. It's been a long hard slog.'

'*A lot of Westerners find the Sai Baba idea a bit difficult to fathom at first. It's a bit of a cultural leap for most of us. How have you coped with it?*'

'Well, at first I was not as committed to it all as Stephen. Then some things happened which made me think very seriously about Sai Baba and the meaning of life in general. I haven't been very well over the last few months and Stephen convinced me to go to Hemma Joshi's house in Edgeware. We were told on the telephone that Sai Baba had appeared to Hemma Joshi and instructed that we were to take a photograph of me when we went to her house. Apparently Sai Baba had said he wanted to bless the picture. I was a bit sceptical about all this but … the most amazing thing happened. We put our picture down on the shrine and suddenly it was covered with tiny, intricate "Om" signs. I couldn't believe it. The photograph was of both of us, Stephen was standing next to me, but the "Om" signs were only on my side of the picture. Literally hundreds of them. Then, as we were leaving, Hemma Joshi said, "Sai Baba will make himself known to you soon."

'I didn't know what this meant but soon found out. I was in hospital a few months later and was just lying there one night when the covers started to move. Then a heavy "body" jumped on the bed and seemed to be running all over it like a cat would. The covers were lifted off me. The night light was on so I can definitely say that no one was in the room. I remembered what Hemma Joshi had said and wondered if this was Sai Baba "making himself known".'

'*So, after this experience, are you more convinced that Sai Baba is behind what's happening at the clinic and elsewhere in the world?*'

'Let me just say that it is very difficult to doubt after the things that have happened to me in the last few months.'

A PERSONAL PERSPECTIVE

I'm driving over to visit the Turoffs. It's a beautiful summer's day. I reflect on the past eight years. It seems more like 80. Everything has changed in my life. Where has that yuppie with the expensive suits, big house, sports car and aeroplane gone? Who was he anyway? What happened to those 12-hour business lunches? And the every-morning hangovers?

I'll tell you what I think might have happened – the yuppie met God, via the Danbury Healing Clinic and Stephen Turoff, and changed his whole outlook on life and way of being in the world.

Heading for Chelmsford, continuing to reflect on those eventful years, I try to count the number of people I've taken to see Stephen for healing, counselling and psychic surgery. It's been a lot of fun. There is often a new experience to be had.

Once I took Jane. Stephen looked at us with his piercing blue eyes and asked, 'Would you like me to manifest the *Atma*?' The *Atma* is God's light. It shines down with varying degrees of intensity into all of us through the top of our head, our crown chakra.

'Yes,' we replied, both looking a little perplexed. Stephen laid Jane down on the operating table with her head at the wall end. He held her ankles and prayed. Standing slightly to one side, I waited, not quite knowing what to expect. After a few seconds, a circle of light began to appear on the wall and got brighter and brighter. Then it just disappeared.

I wondered what was the significance of this event. As if reading my thoughts, Stephen explained, 'I've switched you on.'

'In what way?'

'You'll see.'

Many months later, I'm writing these events down and I am still waiting to see what he meant. But there is one thing of which I am certain from all my experiences with Stephen.

Something will happen that will make it relevant, probably when I least expect it.

I asked Stephen once, 'How can we be sure that only good will come of contact with the other dimensions?'

'Well, as with so many things,' said Stephen, 'the answer is so simple that people often don't take it as seriously as they should. All you have to do is keep your attention focused on God's light. If you are on the correct path, heading Home, this guiding light is always shining like a beacon on the road ahead. The shadow of darkness can only be behind you. Centre your gaze on the light of God and nothing, absolutely nothing, can hurt you.'

8

THE TEMPLE OF HEALING

Health is wealth. Treasure it.

SATHYA SAI BABA

The best way to explain what's going on at the Danbury Healing Clinic is that it is a 'temple of healing'. To give an idea of what happens, I took my video camera there one day, along with some friends who wanted to meet Stephen.

Dr Timothy Ewer is a doctor of medicine practising in New Zealand where, like an increasing number of progressive doctors throughout the world, he offers acupuncture and other energy therapies in addition to orthodox treatment. During the summer of 1996, he was in the UK for training in energy medicine with Harry Oldfield at the School of Electro-Crystal Therapy. He subsequently began offering both electro-crystal therapy (E-CT) and polycontrast interface photography (PIP) at his own general practice in New Zealand. He and his partner, Julie Searle, asked us if they could meet Stephen. Tim wanted to get video footage for PIP research purposes, while Julie was fascinated by what she had heard about the psychic surgeon.

It was a very warm and sunny day when Tim, Julie and I travelled over to Chelmsford. The Miami Hotel was a familiar sight. Arriving at the clinic, the first thing that strikes many people is the queue!

'How long is the wait?' I enquired of Jason.

'Couple of hours,' he answered, smiling apologetically.

We decided on tea and cake in the Miami Hotel restaurant across the courtyard. Afterwards we ambled back and took our seats in the waiting room. I showed some of the photographs to Tim and Julie.

Pointing to one picture, I explained, 'This one is of Sathya Sai Baba. Can you see the ash all over it? As you can see, it's on most of the photos. And on one of the pictures, a red powder called *kumkum* is constantly forming. We're told the ash forms as a gas, liquefies and then turns solid. Interesting, isn't it?'

Tim looked rather sceptical. Like many doctors, he is open-minded about some complementary therapies. However, as a man with a scientific mind and training, he found it hard to accept ash forming on photographs 'from nowhere'. Before I could attempt to explain further, Stephen appeared in the doorway.

'I'm so sorry, everybody,' he said, 'we're running very late today. I'm going as fast as I can. Thank you for your patience.'

A patient caught him in the corridor. 'Mr Turoff, do I need to take anything?'

'Plenty of vitamin G!'

The first time I had heard Stephen say this, I wondered what he meant, as I had never come across vitamin G. When I asked him where to get it, he said, 'It's freely available everywhere. It's God, of course.'

Briefly moving back into the waiting room, Stephen headed straight for Julie and, stooping slightly, stared intently into her eyes for a few seconds. She shuddered a little, then burst gently into tears.

'I know, I know,' he comforted softly and cuddled her for a few moments before moving off back into the operating room. Tim seemed intrigued. Julie let out a sigh of what appeared to be deep and profound release.

As already explained, healing is aimed at the physical, the mental, the emotional and the spiritual self. The spirit team can help Stephen to balance all of these aspects in each person. Often people cry, react angrily or even run out without being seen. Apparently this is all part of the process, the individual experience for each person.

After allowing Tim and Julie to sit and just enjoy the experience for a little while longer, I tried to tell them as much as I could about all the different pictures, signs, idols, gods and so on that occupy the altar and shrine and line the walls at the clinic.

'Having been brought up as a Christian, when I first encountered Hinduism and the other religions represented at Stephen's clinic, I was intrigued by all the elephants, monkeys, many-armed goddesses and so on. I initially believed that these religions had many gods. I have since read that all the major religions of the world worship one supreme being or God. However, each has angels, deities, minor gods and so on which represent *aspects* of the One.'

Tim and Julie appeared to be soaking up the spiritual atmosphere as I continued filming.

'Push, push,' we heard Stephen shouting in the operating room. I learned later that a paraplegic man in a wheelchair was receiving some encouragement to move his toes.

'Good, good.' He had evidently succeeded.

'Do you see the writing on the picture over there?' I continued. The words read 'Love all, serve all' and were handwritten in large orange letters. 'We're told that this is a message which manifested overnight, directly from Sai Baba.'

Before I could continue, Jason called from the hallway, 'Ready, Grant.'

We went into the operating room. Stephen was still in the other room, so I carried on filming and told them some more about the centre and what might happen next.

'This is a picture of Jesus which was manifested by Sai Baba in full view of a large crowd. He was apparently shown the black-and-white picture from the Turin Shroud and asked if it was a true likeness of Jesus. With the devotee holding it, Sai Baba waved his hand over the photograph. An eyewitness told Stephen that the image disappeared. Sai Baba then waved his hand over the photograph a second time. The image reappeared. But the face was slightly different and was now in colour. Sai Baba smiled and said, "This is your Isa." '

In the middle of my explanations, Stephen blustered in. 'Hello again, my friends. Who's first?'

Tim got up on to the bed. When he had made himself comfortable, Stephen threw him a question.

'What do you want?'

Tim thought for a few seconds. 'To be a good doctor and a good healer,' he said, assuredly.

'Be a "God doctor" and you will be a great healer,' said Stephen. 'Where is your problem?'

'My eyes are giving me trouble.'

Stephen, laughing and joking as usual, ignored the eyes, went straight to the lower abdomen and proceeded to carry out psychic surgery in that area. He chatted as he worked.

'Did I tell you, Grant, a woman came over from Denmark recently. She was a quadriplegic. Couldn't move at all. She came on Monday and by Friday she was walking.'

'Oh, that sounds like a good one,' I said. I never know quite what to say when I hear these stories. In a way, I've become so accustomed to miraculous healings that I almost expect them these days. As I continued filming, Stephen grinned from ear to ear and waved at the camera.

'This is supposed to be sensible,' I admonished.

'How can anyone be sensible with Benny Hill looking at them?' he joked.

'I don't look like Benny Hill.'

'Yes you do.'

Suddenly Stephen stared into Tim's eyes. 'Not I, not we, but He! Keep that in your mind.'

Tim seemed fairly comfortable with the whole experience and got up off the table looking pleased. Afterwards he told me, 'It was interesting that he went to the abdomen when I only told him about my eyes, as I do have a problem there. I have no medical or scientific explanation as to how he would know that.'

Tim moved over to where Julie was just getting up from her chair and they kissed.

'I think we'll have to cut that bit out,' I chided.

'Why? That's the best bit,' joked Stephen.

Julie lay down on the bed. She looked a great deal more apprehensive than Tim had done. Once again, Stephen went to the abdomen. His fingers probed the flesh while Julie chatted. 'Ahh! Ohh! Ahh! You wanted sound-effects, didn't you, Grant?' she asked, laughing nervously.

Then Stephen turned to Tim. 'How are you finding your stay?'

'Very good. I'm learning all sorts of wonderful things. And things come together at times, like coming here.'

'Well, if God wants it, it happens!'

'Ohh! Ahh! Ohh!' exclaimed Julie, for real this time. 'You've certainly got the right place. I've never had this kind of massage before.'

Stephen's fingers continued to probe the abdomen. 'This is taking out the rubbish from the emotional centre.'

'Is there a lot of rubbish in there, Stephen?'

'Yes.'

'Thank you. Have you ... ahhh, oh God!' Julie cried out as Stephen removed his fingers with a loud clicking sound.

'Surprised you! Surprised you!' he laughed. 'Fear is like going into a dark room. The first thing you do is switch the light on and the fear goes. The mind is the switch, God is the electricity and the heart is the light. Switch it on.' Stephen paused for a few seconds. 'And that is the truth.' He put his hand back on her abdomen. 'Now we are going to put a little *vibhuti* on it.' He paused again. 'What are you doing in your meditation?'

'Well, I don't do formal meditation, but I do it all the time really. I meditate at the kitchen sink, everywhere.'

'Good. That is the answer I wanted to hear. Your life should be your meditation. Your life should be your prayer. You are not separate from God and God is not separate from you, so why should you need to pray to yourself? Live your prayer.'

'Can I take a picture?' asked Tim as Stephen continued to talk to Julie.

'Of course you can,' he said and paused once more as he looked even more intently at Julie. 'There is no death,' he told her. 'Life and death are like day and night. Summer and winter. In the winter you put an overcoat on and in the summer you take it off.' He clicked Julie's neck, first to the left and then to the right.

'Oh, that feels good. I hold a lot of tension there.'

'Yes. You are a tension little lady.'

We all laughed. Then Julie cried again. Stephen took her hand as she sat up on the table. He clasped it to his chest and stared intently into her eyes once more. There they stood and sat, eyes locked, for what seemed like 10 minutes, but was actually only a couple. 'Good,' said Stephen and, moving over to Tim, stared into his eyes and gave him a hug. Then Stephen told us to have a good day and said he would see us later. Julie blew her nose. Tim smiled. We went back into the waiting room.

I suggested they sit in front of the camera with the shrine and altar behind them while I filmed them. Stephen came out again and was talking to someone. He and the patient are not on the film but the camera recorded what they were saying. The patient had emotional as well as physical difficulties. Stephen was comforting and advising.

'Give your heart to God. Desire nothing else but Him. Tell Him you want nothing but Him, that only His love and light will suffice for you. Be like a child, crying for the mother. Eventually, the mother will answer the child.'

'Stephen, I am so grateful to you,' says the patient. 'You give so much of yourself, every day, for all of these people.'

'I don't own anything, so what can I give you? Nothing. God gives you everything. Try to remember this.'

We left Stephen dealing with the rest of his patients and I chatted to Tim and Julie at some length about their experiences. Both seemed to have enjoyed their visit very much.

Many people come to Stephen at the temple of healing with a 'shopping list' of problems. Some actually write them out in alphabetical order, from 'abscess' through 'piles' to 'vasectomy' and 'warts'. When they go into the operating room, Dr Kahn has no time to explain that they will receive spiritual healing and their treatment must be seen in that light. He sees each patient for only a short time yet a lot is happening. Dr Kahn is communicating spiritually with the patient's higher self, the controlling, guiding aspect of their soul group. Much of their healing has already taken place while they have been waiting in the shrine and altar room. Loved ones from the spirit world are on hand to give support from their side of life.

A number of people have found that they come face to face with themselves when in the presence of Dr Kahn/ Stephen Turoff. Life itself might be a mirror in which we see our own reflection. Perhaps we are given a 'virtual reality' body and let loose in 'EarthWorld', a wonderful simulator in which we each experience the game with our limited senses from our own perspective. Perhaps other people, situations and events provide experiences from which we learn how to play the game better. Might it be that if we bend the rules in one game we will start the next with a physical, mental, emotional or spiritual disadvantage? And after learning all about EarthWorld, perhaps we move on to 'AstralWorld' where there are a number of levels of excellence to be achieved and understood. From an AstralWorld perspective, we may be able to see more of the game and so learn how to help those who are still struggling down in EarthWorld. As we move up the levels, perhaps we will be able to see all the ones below us, but only get glimpses of the next higher one. Do we have eternity to learn that the game is infinite? Whilst in the game, must we have, of necessity, a limited perspective? If we understood the whole game, would we no longer need to play?

I do not pretend to have many answers; for me, it is the questions that are interesting.

9

AVATAR

Love All, Serve All ... 'All' is God.
SATHYA SAI BABA

Sathya Sai Baba has had a great influence on Stephen and his healing mission. As Stephen explains, somewhat surprisingly,

> *God has a 300-year plan! And He's here, now, carrying it out, in human form. Your initial reaction to this news might be slightly sceptical. However, after many years of investigating and personally experiencing the avatar phenomenon that is Sai Baba, I am totally convinced. Convinced that God now walks the Earth in human form. Convinced that this form represents all the previous avatars from Rama to Jesus. Convinced that the triple avatar 300-year plan, predicted by the Upanishads 56 centuries ago, is in progress. Convinced that it is unstoppable. Convinced that we all have a part to play in the plan. Convinced that no soul in human form sees one inch of Sai Baba's robe unless and until he wills it.*

At first I found this all a little strange from my personal perspective – that of a rather lapsed Christian. However, a book called *Sathya Sai Baba and Jesus Christ* by Peter Phipps (Sathya Sai Publications of New Zealand, 1994) helped me to put things in context:

> When Christians hear of a man who has raised the
> dead; constantly heals the sick; can appear in differ-
> ent places at the same time; demonstrates knowl-
> edge of the inner secrets of all people; can speak all
> tongues on earth without having studied languages;
> quotes from all Scriptures of the world without hav-
> ing read them; multiplies food to feed crowds; turns
> water into petrol; produces rings, holy images, medi-
> cines, sweets, out of the air, they should pay atten-
> tion. All the known miracles demonstrated by Jesus
> have been reproduced by Sathya Sai Baba.

Elsewhere in his interesting book, Peter Phipps tells us that
the Sanskrit word for Jesus is *Isa*. The *I* sound means 'mother'
and *sa* means 'divine'. So Jesus means 'mother divine', or
'divine mother', describing the loving, caring concern which
Jesus has for suffering humanity. The same component
sounds may also be written as 'Sai' to have the same meaning.
Baba means 'father'. *Sai Baba*, therefore, means 'divine mother and father' or God.

The coming of God on Earth in human form has been
prophesied in many faiths. The Second Coming of Christ, as
Christians would call it, will see the return of Jesus as a 'thief
in the night'. Buddha said, 'I am not the first Buddha who has
come upon the Earth, nor shall I be the last.' Black Elk, the
great Native American sage who foresaw the coming of the
white man, also told of the coming of a new age, and a mes-
senger of love and understanding who would bring the entire
human race into a circle of love and harmony. Mohammed
told of 'the Guided One' who is to come, who will have great
power, great wisdom and knowledge. He gave a list of 300 features, including a very clear physical description. The Guided
One will, among many other things, be short in stature, live
for 96 years, be highly intelligent, be surrounded by many

followers, have profuse hair, wear red robes, have a mole on the cheek, will give gifts that are light in weight, will tread the path of righteousness and gather the seekers of God around him. Anyone who knows a little about Sai Baba will recognize this description. Mohammed also says that Moslems will not recognize him until nine years before his passing from the Earth. Sai Baba, too, has said that the Moslems will be the last group to receive his message. Nostradamus predicted that, after the Battle of Armageddon, a new saviour will appear to guide the people in the way of truth and peace: 'He who has been awaited for such a long time will not appear in Europe. He will appear in Asia,' and also predicted that Thursday would be his holy day. (It is Sai Baba's holy day.) As for the Battle of Armageddon, the battle to end all battles prophesied in Revelations 16, one idea is that the Second or both World Wars were what is being referred to. The whole of the twentieth century could also be seen as a battle between nations. Another idea is that Armageddon has been going on in the dimensions around the Earth, i.e. on the spirit planes (as well as, perhaps, on the physical plane). A third view is that the battle is yet to come, with great physical upheavals on Earth providing a literal interpretation. As for the 'new saviour', there are similar prophecies in the Book of Revelation and the Jews, of course, are still awaiting the Messiah. Hindus, meanwhile, have a tradition of divine incarnations who come to restore harmony, peace and righteousness among peoples at times of moral and spiritual decline.

Sai Baba himself says,

Call me by any name – Krishna, Allah, Christ. Can't you recognize Me in any Form? Continue your worship of your chosen God along the lines familiar to you and you'll find you are coming near to Me, for all Names and Forms are Mine.

Apparently, the avatar's task of transformation will take three lifetimes or incarnations. One incarnation is already over. The first avatar, Sai Baba of Shirdi, brought central messages of right living (*dharma*) and peace (*shanti*). The current, second avatar brings truth (*sathya*) and the third avatar will bring the most important message, divine love (*prema*), 'love without desire'.

'Swami', as Sai Baba is affectionately known to his people, has attracted Hindus, Moslems, Parsees, Buddhists, Sikhs, Christians, Jews, Jains and a host of other spiritual seekers to his flock – an estimated 150 million people by 1995. But he does not seek converts for a new religion, rather to show us how to better interpret and follow the faith we are familiar with. His simple message of right living, peace, truth and divine love, with no one way of worshipping God being better or worse than any other, has a simplicity which is magnetically attractive.

Sai Baba claims that before he dies in the year 2022, at 96, two thirds of the world will have chosen the path Home. The transformation will usher in a new way of thinking and being for humankind. He tells us that many will doubt this until it is their time not to, but that everything will happen according to its proper time and place and, through the triple avatar incarnation, he *will* achieve his task. To change the thoughts and actions of the vast hordes of humanity, by their own conscious choice, is not, he says, an overnight task. God could, in theory, wave his hand and our tiny world would change instantaneously. But that is not the way it can happen according to God's own Law. God has to incarnate as a human being and communicate with us in a way that we can understand.

If the Sai avatar phenomenon had had such an effect on so many different people, I concluded there must be some substance in it somewhere. Closer investigation revealed an amazing story.

The first avatar, Sai Baba of Shirdi, was born in the area of Hyderabad in the 1840s. Born a Hindu, at an early age he somehow seems to have come under the care of a Moslem fakir, a saintly man, probably a Sufi, who became his first guru. Then he came into the charge of an important government official at Selu, called Gopal Rao, who gave him a broad, if not necessarily traditional education. Before he died, apparently leaving his body by his own yogic power, he pointed to the West and advised the young Sai Baba to travel in that direction in search of his new home.

Sai Baba came to the village of Shirdi in the Bombay presidency and finally settled there permanently in 1872, making the old and rather dilapidated Moslem mosque his home. Some people began to notice he had divine qualities, though most of the villagers thought he was a mad fakir. Traditionally, holy men in India depend on charity for food and other material needs. Sai Baba's needs were few but he did require oil to keep the mosque lights burning through the night, as is both Hindu and Moslem practice. One evening, the shopkeeper who had previously given him oil claimed he had no supplies. He and several villagers thought it a huge joke to see what the mad fakir would do without his oil and followed him back to his mosque. Water jars are kept in mosques for people to wash their feet before entering the sacred area. Sai Baba of Shirdi took water from a jar in full view of the villagers and poured it into his lamps. They continued to burn. He had turned the water into oil! The villagers promptly fell at his feet.

From that time onwards, thousands flocked to Sai Baba as news of his teaching, miracles and instantaneous healings travelled far and wide. He did not need to be in physical proximity to know what was happening to someone and there were many stories of his appearing to protect people when they were many miles from Shirdi. The effect was to draw them to the spiritual way of life. Thousands found their sense of values changing. Some gave up their worldly lives and came to live at Shirdi as close disciples and Sai Baba taught them according to their needs and abilities. Learned religious leaders initially believed him to be illiterate; they found, however, that he could talk about spiritual philosophy and interpret the sacred writings more profoundly and clearly than anyone else.

Sai Baba of Shirdi often proved to devotees that he knew what they were thinking when hundreds of miles away. He appeared whenever and wherever needed. Many testified that he could project himself through space and take any material form he chose. He gave people visions and appeared to them as the particular God-form they worshipped. He granted wishes and appeared to people in dreams. He was able to cast out spirits and cure terrible diseases. He kept a fire burning to ensure a ready supply of sacred ash, which he called *udhi* and used for many miraculous purposes, particularly healing. (*Udhi* is said to be the same substance that the current Sai Baba calls *vibhuti*. This sacred ash is also said to be a symbolic connection between the first and second incarnations.)

By the end of the nineteenth century, despite India's primitive communications at that time, Sai Baba's fame had spread across a huge area. Endless streams of visitors were flowing in. Yet despite all the gifts, the show and the reverence afforded him, Sai Baba continued to beg for his food and when he died, in 1918, he had just enough money to pay for his burial and no more. Just before his death, he said he would come again in eight years. He predicted the time and the place. Eight years later, on 23 November 1926, the second avatar was born.

Sathya Sai Baba was an apparently normal, robust little boy. His popularity with the other village children was ensured by an ability to produce sweets from an empty bag. Apart from avoiding all places where animals were being hurt or slaughtered and bringing home every beggar he could find for his mother to feed, he showed few signs of what was to come.

Then one day he was out walking with friends when he suddenly leapt into the air with a loud cry of pain, holding his right foot, before falling to the ground unconscious. When he came round, he began quoting passages in Sanskrit, far beyond the knowledge of any other 13-year-old. His parents, believing him to be possessed by a demon, called in a exorcist who administered various gruesome 'treatments'. He buried the boy up to his neck in the sand, made cuts in his shaven head with a razor and administered burning lime into the open wounds. Then an acidic substance was poured into Sathya's eyes, which made his face swell beyond recognition. Far from complaining, the boy endured these tortures with good grace. He instructed a relative to fetch certain healing plants and the disfigurements cleared up in no time at all. He later explained that these events were a symbolic demonstration intended to illustrate that neither the pain nor the pleasure of the material, physical illusion we call 'reality' has any effect upon him.

He then provided further evidence of his powers by producing flowers from the air with a wave of his hand. This was too much for his father, who found a hefty stick and faced his son.

'Who are you? What are you?'

'I am Sai Baba!'

His family had no idea what he meant by this, so they fetched the village elders. When they doubted that the boy and the dead holy man were one and the same, Sathya Sai Baba threw the flowers to the ground, whereupon they spelt out his name.

Sai Baba's teaching is either straightforward or deeply philosophical, depending on the audience. He can explain the most difficult mysteries of any sacred text to any expert who comes before him. The underlying principle of his message is that of divine love – love without desire, unconditional and expansive. As he says:

> Start your day with love,
> Spend your day with love,
> Fill your day with love,
> End your day with love.

We are told that the third avatar, Prema Sai Baba, a 'photograph' of whom has already been produced and distributed by Sathya Sai Baba, will devote his whole life to establishing this divine love principle on Earth.

Sathya Sai Baba also teaches that there are other dimensions of reality which operate according to different natural laws. One of these dimensions is the thought dimension. Every single one of our thoughts, whether or not it is voiced or acted upon, is recorded in this dimension for eventual scrutiny. As we think, so we become. My initial reaction to this notion was to panic. If true, most of us are probably in trouble, because none of us, surely, can claim to be absolutely pure in thought, even if we are ostensibly so in word and deed.

Sai Baba has also indicated that this is why he appears to choose the most unlikely people to help in his mission. Those who have the right intentions, whose 'heart is in the right place', are difficult for most of us to distinguish from those who are less well intentioned. Sai Baba, however, tells us that he knows our innermost secrets and our past, present and future. His approach to each individual comes from this all-seeing, all-knowing perspective and his treatment of each of us varies accordingly.

Isaac Tigrett, founder of the Hard Rock Café chain, says that when he meditates, he is taken by Sai Baba on journeys to the thought dimension, together with Phyllis Krystall, author of *Cutting the Ties That Bind* (Turnstone Press, 1982; Weiser, 1993) and *Cutting More Ties That Bind* (Element, 1990; Weiser, 1993), two books which Sai Baba says contain important techniques for releasing ourselves from the chains of our past thoughts, words and actions. Tigrett tells of one time when they were taken to the thought dimension connected with the geographical region of the Soviet Union:

> *As we approached, there was a dark, dense, cloud spreading in all directions. Sai Baba explained that this was the negative energy created by 'a thousand years of the fear of extreme punishment' in this region. Centuries of terrible events in the physical dimension had influenced the thoughts of people which had, in turn, created this black cloud of negative energy. Sai Baba gave us what seemed like huge needles and we all pierced the cloud with them in order to disperse it. A short while later came the collapse of the Soviet Union. It is very difficult to initially comprehend but this is the reality of the enormity of what Sai Baba is doing. He is working constantly, in all the dimensions surrounding the Earth, to create a platform of conditions from which we can launch ourselves into a Golden Age. If He simply put the physical dimension right, He says 'we would be back in the same mess in no time at all'.*

It has become increasingly difficult to avoid the inevitable conclusion that something remarkable does appear to be happening.

In 1994 I went with Stephen to Sai Baba's 69th birthday celebrations in north London. We were accompanied by some
German devotees. When I arrived, one of the women
exclaimed, 'Oh my goodness, I saw you and Stephen last night
in my dream. You were sitting next to each other wearing
white robes.' I had never met this woman before.

At the celebrations, about 1,000 people sat cross-legged
on the floor, men to the right, women to the left. Most people
wore white, the preferred colour of Sai Baba devotees. There
were around three hours of songs and prayers.

Afterwards, many people stayed in the hall and lined
up requesting healing from Stephen. Not having the time to
do much more, he walked along the line touching people on
the forehead. He caught them as they fell backwards, briefly
unconscious, to the floor, then, at the end of one line of about
20 people, he stopped and held his hand in the air without
touching the woman's forehead. A long silence followed as
people waited for something to happen.

'God will visit you tonight,' he said softly. Asia TV had
their cameras rolling throughout and caught all this on film.

Next day the woman's husband rang the clinic and told
Kathy that he had called Asia TV to his house to see the *vibhuti* coming out of the photographs, the walls, everywhere.
Apparently, the woman had not believed in God, but in the
light of the night's events and with ash coming out of every
corner of the house, she was now convinced of his power.

The next year Stephen travelled to Sai Baba's ashram in Puttaparthi, near Bangalore. Although he had been a devotee for
many years, he had never felt the need to actually make the
journey before. God, says Sai Baba, is not a little Indian man
in Puttaparthi. To think so is to go along with the illusion, the
delusion. To think that you need to go to India or become a

Hindu is to miss the point. God is everywhere and everything. On the other hand, Sai Baba has also said that it is sometimes beneficial for 'the coals to come into contact with the burning embers' in order to keep the fire burning brightly. Whatever the reason for the call, Stephen received a message that he was to go and so he went.

The conditions on the ashram are very basic for those used to Western comforts. Nevertheless, Stephen slept on a mattress on the floor, ate the simple vegetarian food, avoided the local water and waited daily in line with thousands of others for a glimpse of Sai Baba. As he explains:

> *My job was to help with sick people. I pushed a lady in a wheelchair to the darshan lines one morning and then joined one of the middle lines myself. A voice in my head said: 'End line one.' I wasn't sure what the message was so I didn't move. Then it came in again, much louder and firmer: 'End line one.' I moved to the end of the line on my right. This was the best I could do to conform to the instruction, but there was no way of knowing which line was going to be allocated number one. The numbers are picked out of a cloth bag so that everything is seen to be fair. Then, to my surprise, the line I was in was allocated 'number one' out of the bag. This meant my line was first in and I was right at the front.*

Sai Baba came out and walked along the lines of people. Stephen knelt up with a note held between both hands. Suddenly, he felt a 'push' from behind and fell uncontrollably forwards. To his horror, his hands landed with a smack on the holy man's feet. Sai Baba smiled, his eyes full of divine love.

'He kept asking me something in a very soft voice. I couldn't hear, so I just handed him the note with my questions on.'

On the note were two questions that Stephen wanted to ask. Sai Baba did not open it but moved on up the line, smiling and acknowledging different people as he went. Some time later, he retired to a building to conduct personal interviews and Stephen decided to walk from the compound into the village to have breakfast. He went to a small hotel and at first was the only person in the dining room. A short while later, a couple of his friends came in and sat with him. Then an Indian gentleman walked in and headed straight for their table. He sat down on the last remaining chair. This was unusual behaviour as all the other tables in the room were unoccupied and none of them had ever seen this man before. The three Westerners acknowledged him politely and continued with their conversation.

Suddenly, the Indian looked straight at Stephen and said, 'You have a lot of kinetic energy. Do you know that your last life was in Calcutta? You were a swami. You have come back into this life for two reasons. The first is "ego", which is nearly dealt with.' He went on to give the second reason, which Stephen prefers to keep private, then said, 'If you can overcome these character traits, you will achieve *mocsha* [liberation] in this lifetime. If you need to know more, I am in room 108.' With that, he stood up and left.

Stephen was amazed. The two subjects were the very same that had been on his note to Sai Baba, the man appeared to know all about him and, to cap it all, was staying in room 108. This is Sai Baba's number and, amongst other things, represents the 108 names of God.

Stephen then had to visit a patient, an American author who lives on the ashram. He walked to her apartment and knocked on the door.

'Ah,' she said. 'I've got a surprise for you. There are two unexpected guests in the other room. They are two elderly Indian ladies, sisters. They have come from Calcutta. They were passing through the ashram and say they decided to pay me a visit. The thing is, Stephen, I don't know them, but I invited them in for tea out of politeness.'

Stephen had never met the ladies either, but made polite conversation over a cup of tea. Then, to his surprise, he started to 'spout poetry'. One of the women began to cry.

'Have I offended you?'

'No. I'm crying for joy because that is the poetry of our master, our swami. He died many years ago in Calcutta.'

This is very strange indeed, thought Stephen. A couple of hours ago I was being told that my last life was as a swami in Calcutta. One of the ladies interrupted his thoughts.

'Our Master was known as "the Pink Swami". He was able to manifest pink lights on photographs. Pink light emanated from his hands and all around his body. He was also a famous poet.'

'That's amazing,' said Stephen. 'Lights manifest on pictures at my clinic and people say they see pink light emanating from my hands and body.'

'Perhaps this is something to think about,' said one of the ladies. With that, they thanked their American host for the tea and left.

This was a lot for Stephen to take in. He went for a long walk to meditate on the day's events and is still unsure what to make of them.

On another occasion I went with Stephen to a house in north London where Sai Baba devotees gather each evening for *bhajans* (religious songs). Stephen was seeking guidance on a particular question and placed a picture of Sai Baba of Shirdi in front of the altar during the prayers. Five minutes later the photograph was literally covered in sacred ash. Stephen had received his answer. No one had been anywhere near the picture.

In August 1995, when Stephen was guest speaker for 1,600 devotees of Sai Baba at Wolverhampton and was waiting to do his speech (extracts of which are on pp.100–2), Sai Baba appeared to him above the shoulders of the man who organized the event, saying, 'This man, Dr Gadhia, is a good man. So are you ... but try harder. Try harder.'

During the October of the same year, Stephen travelled once again to Spain. One Thursday, Sai Baba's day, a group of 40 people were worshipping with him and he was inspired to try feeding milk to a small metal statue. This particular phenomenon was very much in the news at the time. The statue was in the form of Ganesh, an elephant God-aspect which symbolizes 'the moving out of the way of obstacles' in the Hindu religion. Stephen placed a spoonful of milk at the end of the elephant's trunk and all present began the *bhajans*. After about five minutes the milk bubbled and disappeared. Each person present then placed a spoonful of milk in front of Ganesh. Each time it bubbled and disappeared. The volume of milk far exceeded the capacity of the small statue.

Returning home, Stephen found that news of the events had preceded him and he was asked to try the experiment again at the clinic. This time a metal cobra was used and again it 'drank' the milk.

Milk-drinking statues were causing a sensation around the world at that time. Then the phenomenon simply stopped. Stephen believes Sai Baba was making another statement. 'If God had incarnated and wanted to attract our attention it is feasible that He would produce miraculous phenomena which appeared to defy our normal material understanding. In this way He would help us to open our minds to the possibility that there is more to life than we currently understand.'

Another example of this came on 7 August 1996. That morning, in his prayers Stephen asked Sai Baba to 'open the door to my heart'. In the afternoon a French patient arrived.

She had with her a Polaroid camera of the type which develops pictures instantly. To her amazement, as she approached the clinic, she saw something in the clouds above it. Thinking quickly, she raised her camera and took three photographs of the strange image in the sky.

These pictures have to be seen to be believed. The first shows a 'door' made of light in the clouds. The second shows it slightly ajar. The third shows it with a picture of Jesus above it. These Polaroid pictures can be seen at the clinic by anyone who would like to confirm these descriptions for themselves. For Stephen they are just another example of 'a God who listens to our prayers'.

A short while after the Polaroid pictures of the 'door' in the sky were taken by the French patient, a party of Germans arrived for healing. They asked if they could video what went on.

'Of course you can,' agreed Stephen as usual. What happened next, however, wasn't at all usual. The Germans began filming in the waiting room. Later they filmed outside in the hotel grounds. When they played back the film, a bright shining globe, like a second sun, could clearly be seen on the video. This 'sun' moved about above the clinic and burst into a cloud of pink light before reforming as a globe and then bursting into pink light once more. The whole event lasted for a minute or so. The Germans were astounded. So was Stephen when they gave him a copy.

'What do you think is the significance of this?' I asked him.

'Well, I don't know. With the "door" pictures being just before it, I think that the phenomena may be moving outside the clinic as a further illustration of the energy and power that are being manifested here.'

Some friends suggested we might like to put the 'second sun' video on the Internet. Stephen has provided a copy and this is now being arranged. Hopefully, the Internet format will mean that many more people can follow events at the Danbury Healing Clinic as they happen.

Recently, in the early hours of one Monday morning, Stephen awoke from a vivid dream about Sai Baba:

Swami appeared to me in my dream and spoke to me. 'You will be asked to go abroad very soon. And you must go.' I said to Baba that I had such little time. 'Time will be found,' he said. In the dream Sai Baba also materialized something which he then showed me. It was a distinctive gold ring which had nine diamonds in a square black setting. Just as he had shown me the ring, I woke up with an image fixed clearly in my mind.

The next day, Stephen received a phone call from a group of Moslems whose members regularly visit the healing clinic. This group follow a holy man in Pakistan who is in his nineties. The caller said that the holy man had had a stroke and could not move or speak. 'Please can you come with me to Pakistan and administer healing?' Stephen's first thoughts were that he had no time. But then he remembered the previous night's dream and Sai Baba's words, 'And you must go.'

'I quickly consulted the diary,' Stephen told me, 'and found that, if I went Friday evening and came back Sunday afternoon, the trip would just about be feasible. I then had to remind them that I had no visa.'

'No problem' was their reply and so Stephen found himself being picked up and driven to the airport after clinic on the Friday afternoon. When he arrived in Pakistan, he was made very welcome by 60 or so people in the house of the holy man.

After the greetings, I went to the room where the holy man was lying in bed. He was looking very unwell. I walked over to the bed, did my salaams, touched him on the head and asked God to bless him.

There was a short pause. Everyone in the room waited for something to happen.

Within a few minutes the holy man started to speak a few words to his followers. All were amazed at this startling recovery. 'Then he called me over,' continued Stephen, 'and began taking a ring from his finger.'

'God has indicated to me that I should give you this present,' said the holy man. He held the ring out. Stephen took it and immediately recognized it as the ring with nine diamonds that had featured in his dream. The diamonds were set in a square of black onyx.

'I remembered the dream,' says Stephen, 'and thought that it must surely be a gift from Baba. But the ring was too big by far. As I sent out this thought to Baba, the ring shrank immediately to fit my finger perfectly!

'Then I sent out another thought to Baba. Surely I hadn't been called all the way to Pakistan to see this one holy man and get a little gift?'

Stephen soon had what he believes to be his answer. Amongst the many followers of the holy man who were present to witness the miraculous recovery, there were dignitaries and two medical doctors, a husband and wife team. These doctors were so impressed that they asked Stephen how they might serve God better.

'I found myself explaining that the way to serve God is to serve humanity to the best of your ability. I felt that I should suggest that it would be a good idea to open up a medical clinic for the poor where all treatments were free.'

This the doctors agreed to do. Stephen firmly believes that this result was the real purpose behind the dream, the ring and the trek halfway across the world and back in a weekend. 'God truly does seem to work in wonderfully mysterious ways.'

So, what are we to make of all this? Can it be, as claimed by millions, that we are witnessing the long-awaited arrival of God on Earth in human form? There seem to be so many more questions that spring from each answer. I have no desire or intention to offend any person's deeply held conviction or faith. I can only suggest that the interested reader investigates for themselves.

But let me leave you with some of Sai Baba's words:

If you develop love, you do not need to develop anything else.

REFLECTIONS

The name I have answered to for the last 50 years is Stephen Turoff and this is correct for the material world and the society I was born into because name and form represent individuality. Yet to pamper to the needs of our individual name and form and overwhelm them with the toys of the world is not correct. If we are attached to name and form we will be like a child when the toys are taken away from us. We will feel remorse and a sense of loss. I believe that I am here, as Stephen Turoff, to be used as an instrument for God's work. I am part of God, as are everyone and everything else, so all names and forms are mine, as they are yours.

The only attachment we should foster is to God, for He can never be taken from us. Some might say that it is very difficult to achieve non-attachment when we live in such a material society and it is true that non-attachment can only be achieved by knowing who we are. So who are we? I believe that we are all a part of God, that we have all come from God and that we are all on a journey back to God. But more than that, we have none of us ever left God. A fish swims in the sea. The sea is above, below, around and within the fish. In every respect, the fish is part of the sea but it swims along quite happily, not realizing its true nature. Man is the same. He swims through God without realizing his true identity.

God is in our hearts and we are in the heart of God. So, it follows that we can never truly leave Him.

The mind is the only place where we can leave God. Man is the slave of his dreams and desires, for he cannot help but to play the role he has himself created. In the play of life, however, it is essential to take time off to speak to the producer and we can do this through prayer. Prayer can move mountains if we reach that level of superconsciousness where we know, without doubt, our true nature.

We must first learn to control our own desires. When we master them, then no harm can befall us. We have to sharpen our intellect and use that wonderful God-given imaginative capability to conceive God in all his glory. We may think that our imagination has caused us all sorts of problems, with our many desires and dreams of worldly riches. We have all had many bad thoughts and have committed what our conscience tells us are bad actions. How do we proceed from here? Unless we are willing to stand back from the entanglement of the world, knowing full well that it is a play which we ourselves have created for the pleasure of the lower instincts, we are in danger of losing sight of the true reason for our existence. We should use this lifetime in devotion to God. Through service and sacrifice, we can clear the dead wood away and plant anew the seeds of good deeds. Selfless service will take root and produce the fruits of our labour.

You might say, 'This is all very well in theory, but how do I still my mind, which wants to throw up all manner of past and future problems to distract and attach me to either yesterday or tomorrow?' I would respond by saying that the past is gone and the future is uncertain. And when tomorrow comes, it is today. So now is the moment. Today is ours. See good, do good, be good, *now*.

All our pains and heartaches arise because of the failure to understand the workings of the mind. If we turn our minds towards God, we have the appropriate tool for liberation. Keep the mind dwelling only on the toys of Earth and it will become the means of bondage. Our primary aim should be to turn our minds to God.

If you were walking down a dark lane at night towards your house, you would find yourself walking more quickly than normal because of an inner fear of the darkness. When you reached your house, what would be the first thing you would do? You would open the door and put the light on. Then, after shutting the door and removing your coat, you would begin to feel safe and at ease. To achieve this feeling, all you would have done is to switch the light on. The mind is the switch, God is the electricity and the heart is the light. Use the switch of your mind so that the electricity of God can flow through you and turn on the light in your heart.

I have been asked how it is we can know whether God hears our prayers when it sometimes seems that the problems of the world continue to trouble us even if we have prayed long and hard for a solution. Should we complain about our troubles and that God has not ended them immediately for us? Should we think He has shown us no compassion or understanding? I would first ask, 'What compassion or under-standing have we given God?' When you were five years old, you would play with your friends and at times you would fall and hurt yourself. You would sob and cry out aloud until your mother came running to you. She would pick you up, rub your knee and comfort you until the tears were all dried up and you would again begin to play with your friends. You have the appropriate instrument to call God, just as you had the appro-priate instrument to call your mother. Keep crying for the Lord, for He will hear you. He will send you signs and sym-bols to let you know that He has heard your cry. But do not be happy with just the toys. Tell God, 'The only thing that will stop me crying is Oneness with You.'

Merely uttering the name of God is not enough. We can-not be certain to catch the Lord's attention with mere words. Action speaks louder than words. Service, duty, charity and, above all, love should be the mainstays of our lives. Service with love, duty with love, charity with love should be every-day manifestations of our embodiment of love. We should cite the name of God with love as we venture throughout the day. We should try to practise the meditation of divine vision, which is seeing God in everything, everywhere, all the time. We should be continually rendering some kind of service to those who are less fortunate than ourselves. When we are engrossed in prayer and thinking only of our own unhappiness and our own salvation, we should stop and give a thought to those who are worse off than ourselves.

The smallest action has value. Just as a stone hitting the tranquil pool will send ripples cascading outwardly, so an action will have the same effect for good or evil. Always the thought first, then the action will follow. If all thought and actions are dedicated to God, there can only be good consequences for all. This in turn gives the servant good feelings and leads him on to greater heights of awareness through his conscious development. The more we become 'self-realized', the more we will wish to serve God. As we venture through life, we are attracted by those who think on the same wavelength as ourselves, and we find comfort in our mutual knowledge and appreciation of God.

However, we also come across the negative people who try at every turn to discredit us and our knowledge. These are the people we must work harder upon. Our interaction with people affects our karma. A farmer spends much time getting ready the field in which he is to plant his seed. The field will contain only one sort of seed, so the farmer is certain to reap only one type of harvest. If we plant only good seeds in this life, so in the next life we will reap the results. We should recognize the existence of the moral law as governing all action. Therefore we should not lose sight of our objective until there is no more sowing or reaping and freedom has been reached.

God's grace is won by suffering only – and I do not mean just suffering of material substance. Until your heart tears away from the centre of self-indulgence and accepts its moral responsibility to humanity, it cannot hope to undergo the spiritual change which will lead on towards self-realization. Think of all the seeds you have sown today; if you have planted a thought deep into someone's consciousness, you will shortly see its result. But the responsibility is yours, for in life we are all gardeners, ever sowing and reaping the fruits of our actions.

God has planted the seed of life deep into our hearts; within the seed is God's word for the cultivation of mankind. ('Of My Self, I have given thee.') A good gardener will tell you how deep a certain seed should be planted, when to water it and how much to feed it. He will tend the seed with care, taking away any weeds that grow around the young seedling. God has made us all gardeners of His seed. The water of knowledge is necessary for its growth, as well as perseverance in clearness of thought. We must not get entangled in the weeds of materialism, otherwise the growth of the seed will be strangled by the distractions of this world.

It is important to control our bad habits. Our success in achieving a spiritual way of life is hastened or delayed by our habits. It is no use getting up in the morning and praying, or thinking to work harder, for more money. It is in the way that we are steadfast in our mental habits that helps us achieve spiritual success. Prayer is a good habit only if it is used in talking to the Lord for the benefit of others and not just for ourselves.

In all religious activities people are drawn together because of their common faith and beliefs. Their minds are focused upon their feelings of unity with God and with one another. A man who truly believes in his faith, and who has his heart filled with God's love, will live his life in unity with all of humanity. He will treat both believers and unbelievers as his brothers and sisters, for a man who has reached self-realization knows no boundaries or limitation.

If asked, 'What is your religion?' I believe each of us should answer: 'There is only one God, the God of humanity, only one religion, the religion of love. Truth is my religion, service my worship, the world my family. I strive to practise the principle of "no limitation" and "no discrimination between colour or creed".' We should not be drawn into a debate about which religion is 'best'. I believe we should strive to respect all religions but follow our own with the utmost vigour. Religion is about living our lives according to certain principles. All religions encourage us to be honest, truthful, helpful, sincere and of service to humanity whilst avoiding harm to others. Good-hearted love and service, that is real religion.

Our attachment should be to truth because only truth can set us free. Everything has something of God; man is the highest earthly manifestation of His divine love. We should see God in everything. But our quest should not stop there. We should seek higher and higher states of consciousness. The world is our temple and we should treat everyone and everything in it as we would wish to be treated.

Love all, serve all ... Sai Ram.

STEPHEN TUROFF

POSTSCRIPT

Throughout my eight-year investigation into the work of Stephen Turoff, I have personally seen what appeared to be an image of Dr Kahn smiling at us on Harry Oldfield's PIP machine, sensed the presence of spirit beings, taken part in table-moving and 'sittings', been present during many apparently successful psychic surgery operations, witnessed inexplicable manifestations of sacred ash and sweet-scented oil and experienced many indirect 'proofs' ranging from lights appearing on photographs taken by others to audio tapes recording the voices of 'dead' people and the reports of the numerous patients who have been kind enough to tell me the details of what happened to them.

I had not, however, had any direct personal revelations, visions or experiences without being in the presence of Stephen Turoff or at his clinic. This changed in early August 1996, when I visited my publishers in London to discuss this book.

Their offices are in a modern building with long open landings which are arranged around a central atrium. Many offices have windows which look out onto the landings and during the meeting I was looking out in that direction. Suddenly, a short figure with a huge mop of black crinkly hair and a long orange robe walked briefly along the landing. I rose from my chair in disbelief. It was unmistakably Sathya Sai Baba – who was in India at the time. This was not an apparition; it was a solid body walking in the normal way.

I am aware that for some, this admission will damage my credibility beyond recovery. But please be assured that I sincerely believe it to be the truth.

On reflection, I concluded that this event was a confirmation that I was in the right place. You will have to make of it what you will.

GRANT SOLOMON